OVERCOMING MILD TRAUMATIC BRAIN INJURY AND POST-CONCUSSION SYMPTOMS

A self-help guide using evidence-based techniques

Nigel S. King

D0370219

ROBINSON

Dr Nigel King is a Consultant Clinical Neuropsychologist specializing in head injury and trauma. He is a world-renowned authority on mild traumatic brain injury and post-concussion symptoms and regularly speaks at national and international conferences on these subjects. He is also: a Fellow of Harris Manchester College, University of Oxford; the Head of Clinical Neuropsychology at the Community Head Injury Service, Aylesbury, UK; a Clinical Tutor at the Oxford Institute of Clinical Psychology Training; and a Full Registrant on the British Psychological Society's Specialist Register of Clinical Neuropsychologists. He has published widely in internationally refereed journals on mild traumatic brain injury and post-concussion symptoms, and he co-edited *Psychological Approaches to Rehabilitation after Traumatic Brain Injury* – a book commissioned by the British Psychological Society.

His National Health Service position includes the provision of specialist neuropsychological treatment for all patients in the county of Buckinghamshire with traumatic brain injury. His Clinical Tutor position includes responsibilities for the Clinical Neuropsychology Module and the Expert Witness & Court Work teaching on the Oxford Doctoral Course in Clinical Psychology. His prior experience has been across a broad range of in-patient and outpatient settings for patients with both neurological and mental health problems. In addition to Dr King's National Health Service work he regularly conducts medicolegal assessments on behalf of lawyers acting for claimants or defendants, or as a single joint expert.

The aim of the **Overcoming** series is to enable people with a range of common problems and disorders to take control of their own recovery programme.

Each title, with its specially tailored programme, is devised by a practising clinician using the latest techniques of cognitive behavioural therapy – techniques which have been shown to be highly effective in changing the way patients think about themselves and their problems.

Many books in the Overcoming series are recommended by the UK Department of Health under the Books on Prescription scheme.

Please note that all of the case studies in this book are fictionalized composites of patients I have seen, or have been known to me. Any resemblances to real life cases are therefore entirely coincidental.

ROBINSON

First published in Great Britain in 2015 by Robinson

Copyright © Nigel S. King, 2015

3 5 7 9 10 8 6 4 2

Important Note
This book is not intended as a substitute for medical advice or treatment. Any person with a condition requiring medical attention should consult a qualified medical practitioner or suitable therapist.

A CIP catalogue record for this book
is available from the British Library.

ISBN: 978-1-47213-609-1 (paperback)
ISBN: 978-1-47213-610-7 (ebook)

Typeset in Bembo by Initial Typesetting Services, Edinburgh

Printed and bound by Clays Ltd, Elcograf S.p.A.

Papers used by Robinson are from well-managed forests and other responsible sources

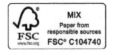

Robinson
An imprint of
Little, Brown Book Group
Carmelite House
50 Victoria Embankment
London EC4Y 0DZ

An Hachette UK Company
www.hachette.co.uk
www.improvementzone.co.uk

For Mum & Dad, Paul, Emma, Ade and Rachel

Acknowledgements

With huge thanks to Sandra Barton, Alice Coates, Russell Forster and Derick Wade for their insightful and helpful comments on the first draft of the book, and equally huge thanks to Angela Fox for her invaluable administrative support.

Acknowledgments

Contents

Foreword

The approach this book takes in attempting to help you overcome your problems with mild traumatic brain injury is a 'cognitive behavioural' one. A brief account of the history of this form of intervention might be useful and encouraging. In the 1950s and '60s a set of therapeutic techniques was developed, collectively termed 'behaviour therapy'. These techniques shared two basic features. First, they aimed to remove symptoms (such as anxiety) by dealing with those symptoms themselves, rather than their deep-seated underlying historical causes (traditionally the focus of psychoanalysis, the approach developed by Sigmund Freud and his associates). Second, they were scientifically based, in the sense that they used techniques derived from what laboratory psychologists were finding out about the mechanisms of learning, and they put these techniques to scientific test. The area where behaviour therapy initially proved to be of most value was in the treatment of anxiety disorders, especially specific phobias (such as extreme fear of animals or heights) and agoraphobia, both notoriously difficult to treat using conventional psychotherapies.

After an initial flush of enthusiasm, discontent with behaviour therapy grew. There were a number of reasons for this. An important concern was the fact that behaviour therapy did not deal with the internal thoughts that were so obviously central to the distress that many patients were experiencing. In particular, behaviour therapy proved inadequate when it came to the treatment of depression. In the late 1960s and early 1970s a treatment for depression was developed called 'cognitive therapy'. The pioneer in this enterprise was an American psychiatrist, Professor Aaron T. Beck. He developed a theory of depression which emphasized the importance of people's depressed styles of thinking, and, on the basis of this theory, he specified a new form of therapy. It would not be an exaggeration to say that Beck's work has changed the nature of psychotherapy, not just for depression but for a range of psychological problems.

The techniques introduced by Beck have been merged with the techniques developed earlier by the behaviour therapists to produce a therapeutic approach which has come to be known as 'cognitive behavioural therapy' (or CBT). This therapy has been subjected to the strictest scientific testing and has been found to be highly successful for a significant proportion of cases of depression. However, it has now become clear that specific patterns of disturbed thinking are associated with a wide range of psychological problems, not just depression, and that the treatments which deal with these are highly effective. So, effective cognitive behavioural treatments have been developed for a range of anxiety disorders, such as panic disorder, Generalised Anxiety Disorder, specific phobias, social phobia, obsessive compulsive disorders, and hypochondriasis (health anxiety), as well as for other conditions such as drug addictions, and eating disorders like bulimia nervosa. Indeed, cognitive behavioural techniques have been found to have an application beyond the narrow categories of psychological disorders. They have been applied effectively, for example, to helping people with low self-esteem, those with weight problems, couples with marital difficulties, as well as those who wish to give up smoking or deal with drinking problems.

The current addition to the Overcoming series concerns *mild traumatic brain injury and post-concussion symptoms*. Such injuries commonly cause difficulties in thinking, emotion, and physical health. Much of this book concerns how sufferers can use cognitive behavioural techniques to cope with such difficulties. This book introduces to the series a new concept, namely 'cognitive rehabilitation'. Such rehabilitation requires the development of a detailed understanding of a person's individual strengths and weaknesses in their thinking skills and finding practical ways of achieving optimal functioning. Three critical principles are outlined: reducing mental load, managing mood, and accepting limitation and findings ways to get around difficulties; and for each, details are provided of how these principles can be used to improve the lives of those suffering from brain injury and post-concussion symptoms. While appropriate clinical investigation and treatment is essential, collectively, the cognitive behavioural techniques outlined and the cognitive rehabilitation principles described in this self-help manual will be invaluable tools to those suffering mild traumatic brain injury and post-concussion symptoms, as well as those living with them and caring for them.

Although effective CBT treatments have been developed for a wide range of disorders and problems, these treatments are not widely available; and, when people try on their own to help themselves, they often, inadvertently, do things which make matters worse. Over the past two decades, the community of cognitive behavioural therapists has responded to this situation. What they have done is to take the principles and techniques of specific cognitive behavioural therapies for particular problems, of proven effectiveness, and present them in manuals which people can read and apply themselves. These manuals specify a systematic programme of treatment which the person works through to overcome their difficulties. In this way, cognitive behavioural therapeutic techniques of established value are being made available on the widest possible basis.

The use of self-help manuals is never going to replace the need for therapists. Many people with emotional and behavioural problems will need the help of a trained therapist. It is also the case that, despite the widespread success of cognitive behavioural therapy, some people will not respond to it and will need one of the other treatments available. Nevertheless, although research on the use of these self-help manuals is at an early stage, the work done to date indicates that for a great many people such a manual is sufficient for them to overcome their problems without professional help. Sadly, many people suffer on their own for years. Sometimes they feel reluctant to seek help without first making a serious effort to manage on their own. Sometimes they feel too awkward or even ashamed to ask for help. Sometimes appropriate help is not forthcoming despite their efforts to find it. For many of these people the cognitive behavioural self-help manual will provide a lifeline to a better future.

Professor Peter J. Cooper,
University of Reading, 2015

Important Background Information

'No head injury is too trivial to ignore.'

Hippocrates, 460–377 BC

If you have suffered a 'mild traumatic brain injury' (MTBI) or 'mild head injury' (MHI) you may be experiencing difficulties with post-concussion symptoms (PCS). These can include headaches, dizziness, fatigue, irritability, sleep disturbance, reduced day-to-day memory, poor concentration, taking longer to think, 'muzzy'-headedness, depression, anxiety, tinnitus, blurred or double vision, sensitivity to light or noise, frustration, nausea, restlessness and sensitivity to alcohol. When they persist beyond a few months or are particularly severe they are sometimes called post-concussion syndrome. In such circumstances the 'mild' head injury may feel anything but mild. This is particularly true if large areas of your day-to-day life are affected. Unfortunately this is not at all uncommon for those with prolonged symptoms.

Different Explanations

When people have post-concussion symptoms their difficulties can be made worse by the different explanations they may get for their persisting problems. This usually involves receiving contradictory opinions about the degree to which ongoing PCS are caused by brain-injury factors or other factors. Brain-injury factors could include any physical damage to the brain itself or changes in the ways that 'chemical messages' in the brain work. The 'other' factors might include the emotional impact of the event that caused the injury, stressful life events not directly related to the injury, ongoing pain, ongoing sleep disturbance or stressful life events that have happened since the injury.

Indeed, there is some evidence that different types of clinician tend to favour different types of explanation for persisting post-concussion symptoms. Also, many problems experienced after mild traumatic brain injury are very similar to those experienced by patients with very severe brain injuries – for example with thinking skills like day-to-day memory, concentration, speed of thinking, mental stamina or multi-tasking. It is therefore unsurprising that someone with a MTBI might easily think that they have suffered a very substantial brain injury.

Different Outcomes

Further problems can arise because the vast majority of mild traumatic brain-injury patients make a complete recovery within the first few weeks or months. This can make it particularly difficult to make sense of prolonged post-concussion symptoms. Also, many people are aware that head injuries, even mild ones, can have very serious and sometimes life-threatening complications. Unfortunately there are a small number of famous people who have experienced these very rare complications, which makes this fact very well-known. Unsurprisingly this can raise further concerns about whether a mild traumatic brain injury has been properly assessed or treated. It is less well known, however, that it is usually entirely normal for those with MTBI not to receive a brain scan as part of their initial examination. Also, the very rare complications normally only occur within the first few hours, days or weeks, rather than months after an injury. Nonetheless if PCS are prolonged it can easily feel like the injury has never been fully assessed and that something serious may have been missed.

Getting the Right Kind of Help

These complicating factors can make it very difficult to find the right kind of help. Patients can easily feel like they are being 'pushed from pillar to post' when trying to find services that can assist with their problems. On top of all of this, there is a distinct lack of good, science-based information for patients about the best ways to manage PCS. It is therefore very common for those who experience prolonged difficulties to find their situation extremely confusing, frustrating and stressful.

This Book

I have spent my entire career treating patients with mild traumatic brain injury and researching post-concussion symptoms, and I have become increasingly aware of the absence of information that is practical, science-based and patient-focused. Over the years I have produced a large number of self-help information sheets for my patients and have also had quite a large number of scientific papers published in medical journals and books. Having had this rare opportunity to work in the area for so long and having already written on many aspects of it, it therefore seemed right for me to take some personal responsibility for 'plugging this gap'.

This book weaves together a great deal of what I have written about in different settings to provide, in one place, a summary of the most useful practical knowledge in this area. It hopefully clarifies at least some of the complex issues for those who suffer with prolonged problems and provides practical, evidence-based self-help guidance for managing MTBI difficulties.

How to Use the Book

The book is divided into four sections.

Section 1 summarizes and explains mild traumatic brain injury, post-concussion symptoms and the most up-to-date ways of understanding prolonged problems. **This section should be read all the way through to best help**

4

understand the area because it is definitely true that 'knowledge is power' when it comes to persisting PCS.

Section 2 summarizes some of the most helpful self-help strategies for a wide range of thinking-based, emotional and physical difficulties that can be experienced after a MTBI. They stem from two main ways of understanding problems:

1. Cognitive rehabilitation approaches – which look at how best to understand and manage changes in our thinking abilities – such as memory, concentration and multi-tasking skills.
2. Cognitive behavioural approaches – which look at the ways in which our thoughts, feelings, actions and physical reactions relate to each other.

There is some overlap across these strategies (as you will see if you read the whole book!) and it is rare for someone to experience all of the problems covered. **There is a short introduction to both these approaches. These are designed to be read by everyone. The strategies that follow are to be read on a 'pick and choose' basis depending on the specific areas that are relevant to the reader.**

Section 3 provides short summaries of some of the self-help strategies outlined in Section 2. These summaries can be scanned or photocopied and used as easy-to-read information sheets. They contain the information that is most often needed by other people if they are going to be involved in helping you manage your PCS. You may therefore want to give these to family, friends or colleagues who want to understand some of the problems encountered after a MTBI.

Section 4 provides a short conclusion of what is covered in the book by revisiting the key 'take home messages'. It also highlights additional useful resources.

Important Health Warning

It is vitally important to recognize that many of the strategies in this book work best with the help of an appropriately trained clinician. If they do not work as self-help techniques this does not mean that they can never work for you. It may just mean that professional help from a clinician is needed for them to be effective. Therefore do not hesitate in getting such help if some of them do not work for you.

The Key 'Take Home Messages'

There are eight key 'take home messages' that I hope you take away from this book.

1. *The Brain Is Incredibly Complicated*
   The brain is the most complicated thing in the universe and although we know a great deal about how it works there is still a huge amount that we do not understand about it.

2. *Mild Traumatic Brain Injury Does Not Always Have 'Mild' Consequences*

   If you have suffered a mild traumatic brain injury and are experiencing ongoing post-concussion symptoms then the term 'mild' is likely to be a very inaccurate way of describing your problems. Your symptoms may well affect many areas of your life and may severely limit what you are able to do.

3. *Same Symptoms, Different Causes and Different Explanations*

   Post-concussion symptoms and many problems after mild traumatic brain injury can be identical to those caused by other factors – including stress, pain, physical difficulties, sleep disturbance, emotional difficulties and severe brain injury. This may make it very difficult to understand your problems. This is made worse by the differing explanations you may receive from different clinicians.

   Some may tell you that your ongoing problems are caused by your brain injury. Others may say they are caused by emotional and psychological factors. Still others may believe that both brain injury and emotional factors are at work. These opinions may well be stated very confidently even though they are very different! Clearly this will not help you understand your problems. In many ways, however, the more that your difficulties are actually caused by non-brain injury factors the better it is. This is because there will be a greater chance that they may be fully overcome.

4. *Stand Back from Your Problems to 'See the Wood for the Trees'*

Regardless of the extent to which your symptoms are caused by brain injury or non-brain injury factors, the best place to start to understand them is to write a list of all the different things that might contribute to your current symptoms. This will help start the process of standing back from your problems to 'see the wood from the trees' and to gain a bird's-eye view of your difficulties.

The list might include thinking difficulties such as: reduced multi-tasking abilities; mental fatigue; poor concentration; slower thinking speed; short-term memory deficits; reduced mental stamina; troubles with planning; or difficulties with problem solving. They might also include emotional difficulties such as: post-traumatic stress; anxieties surrounding a compensation claim or other legal proceedings; worries about family or work tasks; perfectionism; anger or irritability; low mood; driving anxiety; or concerns about the head injury itself. Additional difficulties may involve physical problems. These might include: poorer sleep; headaches; tiredness; pain; sensitivity to light or noise; dizziness; or tinnitus.

5. *Create a Full Personalized Explanation of Your Specific Problems*

A vital step may then be to create a full, personalized explanation of your specific problems. Often this will be in the form of a 'Box Diagram' for your own condition. This will help highlight what vicious cycles have developed over time and which ones are maintaining your symptoms or making them worse. This can be the most important step in overcoming PCS as 'knowledge is power' when it comes to managing MTBI.

6. *Cognitive Behavioural and Cognitive Rehabilitation Strategies*

The most effective strategies for tackling each of the 'boxes' will probably come from cognitive rehabilitation or cognitive behavioural therapy (CBT) approaches. The cognitive rehabilitation strategies that work best are the 'external' ones rather than 'brain training' exercises. These involve finding practical ways to get around the different types of thinking difficulties you may have. The key principles involved are:

a) understanding your own individual cognitive strengths and weaknesses;

b) identifying only one new strategy to try at any one time and being certain that this is the one *you* want as *your* goal;

c) acknowledging that until a new strategy has become a habit, it can take some effort to keep going with it. Usually after 4–8 weeks of consistent practice it will become a routine part of your daily life.

The cognitive behavioural approaches involve understanding the powerful idea that feelings, thoughts, actions and bodily sensations do not just interact with each other in one direction – they interact in a combination of all directions. CBT then involves identifying vicious cycles caused by these different factors 'playing off each other' and using techniques to reverse them so they become 'virtuous cycles'.

7. *Do Not Worry if You Cannot Find Helpful Strategies on Your Own*
    You should not worry if you find it difficult to create your own 'Box Diagram' or if you are unable to find effective strategies on your own. It is very common for those with persisting post-concussion symptoms to need the help of a clinician especially if: it is difficult to stand back from the problems; it is difficult to know where to start because things seem overwhelming; or some of the solutions seem to 'oppose each other'. An example of 'opposing' strategies would be when your diary really helps you with your memory difficulties but robs you of the chance to test out whether your memory is in fact better than you think it is or to challenge negative thoughts about

how bad it would be if you do experience memory 'failures'.

Do not hesitate to keep looking for a clinician with experience in mild traumatic brain injury who can provide the right kind of help for you. Unfortunately this may involve some persistence as you may not always find the right kind of help the first time around. The right kind of professional can often be a Clinical Neuropsychologist but this will not always be the case.

8. *The Number of Strategies is Limitless so be Creative!*
Any number of strategies can be used to creatively tackle each of your 'boxes' to make your own 'virtuous cycles' and overcome your PCS to the greatest possible degree. The book only lists the most frequently used ones. Strategies that help any individual are only really limited by their own understanding of what is causing their problems and their imagination to invent ways around them. So be creative!

I very much hope that if you are experiencing prolonged post-concussion symptoms the book will provide help, hope and understanding for what can be a highly disabling and misunderstood condition.

Section 1

This section should be read all the way through to best understand mild traumatic brain injury because, as previously mentioned, 'knowledge is power' when it comes to persisting post-concussion symptoms.

The Human Brain

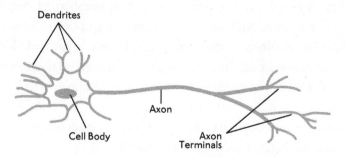

The human brain is probably the most complicated thing in the universe. It weighs about 3 lbs (1.4 kg) and has the texture of toothpaste. It is made up of 50–100 billion nerve cells called neurons as well as 500–1,000 billion other cells. Neurons have a cell body with lots of branches coming off them called dendrites. They also have long tails called axons which are insulated by a sheath (myelin sheath). At the end of the axons are small branches called terminal branches.

All of these branches form connections with other neurons, making a vast number of connections throughout the brain.

How Messages Are Sent

Messages are sent through these neurons by incredibly quick electrical charges, which are relayed by incredibly quick chemical reactions. Different neurons can have different types of chemical transmitters that allow the messages to be passed from neuron to neuron. You may have heard of some of these – serotonin, noradrenaline, dopamine, etc. So throughout your life, even when you are sleeping, the brain is sending billions of messages through these neurons at extremely high speeds through vast numbers of chemical reactions. Messages are also sent to and from the brain by the neurons in the spinal cord in our backs and along the nerves in our bodies. These messages allow us to move our bodies and experience feeling. For example, when you decide to move your hand, messages from the brain travel down the neurons in your spinal cord through to the nerves in your hand, which make the muscles move.

Different Parts of the Brain

On the surface of the brain the outer layer is about a quarter of an inch deep and is called the cortex. It is made up of a large concentration of neuron cell bodies, which gives it a grey-looking colour under the microscope. This is where the phrase 'using your grey matter' comes from. Below this area are a large number of neuron tails (axons). These act as connectors between different parts of the cortex, a bit like a very complicated telephone wiring system. They are white in colour under the microscope.

Although the brain is extremely complicated we do know that different areas have different responsibilities. In most people, the left-hand side of the brain generally controls language, logical thinking, awareness of time and most things to do with written and spoken communication. The right-hand side of the brain is responsible for analysing visual information and for our experiences of three-dimensional space, artistic impression and 'intuition'. The main areas of the brain are also divided into different lobes which have different responsibilities although they all work in partnership with each other:

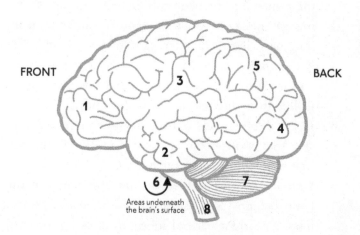

1. *Frontal Lobe* – The front part of the brain is responsible for planning, self-awareness, monitoring, coming up

with ideas and putting ideas into action. These are often termed executive functions. There is an area on the left-hand side of the frontal area (Broca's area) that is responsible for finding the words and sentences we need when we speak or write.

2. *Temporal Lobe* – These are the areas on the lower sides of the brain. The left temporal lobe normally controls the memory of verbal information, i.e. information that is written or spoken. The right temporal lobe is normally responsible for visual and spatial memory, i.e. information to do with vision and space. There is also an area towards the back of the left temporal area (Wernicke's area) that is responsible for understanding language.

3. *Sensory and Motor Strips* – There is a strip just behind the frontal lobe that controls the sending and receiving of messages about movements in your arms, shoulders, legs and other parts of your body. This is the motor strip. Immediately behind this is the sensory strip, which receives and sends messages of feeling from different parts of your body.

4. *Occipital Lobe* – At the back of the brain there is an area that controls the analysis of visual information sent from your eyes to the brain.

5. *Parietal Lobe* – The area on the upper side of the brain behind the sensory strip is called the parietal lobe. The right parietal lobe processes information to do with space and the awareness of your body movements.

6. *Sub-cortical areas* – These are the areas of the brain underneath the cortical area. They are involved with controlling feelings, emotions, pain, temperature, movement and general levels of alertness.

7. *Cerebellum* – This large part of the brain at the back controls the coordination of movements that we decide to make.

8. *Brain Stem* – This area of the brain just above the top of the spinal cord controls our basic life-support systems like breathing, swallowing and how conscious we are.

Traumatic Brain Injury

One of the most important things to know about traumatic brain injury (TBI) is that all head injuries are different and each person's response to a head injury is different. There is therefore no such thing as a 'typical head injury'.

Measuring the Severity of Traumatic Brain Injury

The terms 'traumatic brain injury' or 'head injury' cover a very broad range of injuries. They include mild traumatic brain injury, which normally involves no measurable brain damage and complete recovery within a few days, through to extremely severe brain damage resulting in permanent coma or death. Some of the best ways to measure the severity of a head injury include:

1. the length of any unconsciousness associated with the injury;

2. the period of time between suffering the injury and regaining moment-by-moment memory for events – post-traumatic amnesia;

3. the results of any neurological investigations that may have been necessary, e.g. CT or MRI brain scans (these are, however, rarely required after most mild head injuries);

4. the depth of any changes in consciousness immediately after the injury. This is often measured by the Glasgow Coma Scale (GCS) score, where the total from the three sections runs from 3 (the most deeply unconscious you can be) to 15 (full consciousness and full orientation):

Glasgow Coma Scale

Symptom	Score
Opens eyes on their own	4
Opens eyes when asked to in a loud voice	3
Opens eyes to pain	2
Does not open eyes	1
Carries on a conversation correctly and tells the examiner where they are and the year and the month	5
Seems confused or disorientated	4
Talks so the examiner can understand them but makes no sense	3
Makes sounds that examiner can't understand	2
Makes no noise	1

Follows simple commands	6
Pulls examiner's hand away on painful stimuli	5
Pulls a part of his or her body away on painful stimuli	4
Flexes body inappropriately to pain	3
Decerebrate posture – head and neck arched backwards, arms and legs held straight out and toes pointed downwards	2
Has no motor response to pain	1

Source: G. Teasdale and B. Jennett, 'Assessment of coma and impaired consciousness', *Lancet*, 2 (1974), 81–4.

Generally speaking the longer the period of unconsciousness, the greater the depth of unconsciousness; and the longer the length of post-traumatic amnesia, the more severe the head injury is likely to be.

Classifications of Head-injury Severity

A very crude assessment of the severity of a head injury would be:

- *'Mild or moderate head injury'* when post-traumatic amnesia is less than twenty-four hours and/or there is an initial Glasgow Coma Scale score of 13–15.

- *'Severe head injury'* when post-traumatic amnesia is between one to seven days and/or there is an initial GCS of 9–12.

- *'Very severe head injury'* when post-traumatic amnesia

19

is more than seven days and/or there is an initial GCS of 8 or less.

It should be recognized, however, that these are very much 'rough rule of thumb' indicators of injury severity and that there are huge variations in outcome even within these categories. For example, whilst many who sustain a 'very severe' injury will be left with at least some significant and permanent brain damage, some will ultimately make a complete recovery. As we will see later on, the opposite can also be true – the vast majority with a mild or moderate injury will make a complete recovery but a small number may be left with prolonged or permanent difficulties.

Damage to the Brain after Severe and Very Severe Injuries

After a severe or very severe traumatic brain injury, damage to the brain can occur due to:

1. the brain being bruised (contusion);
2. nerve cells (neurons) being damaged or destroyed;
3. connections between nerve cells being damaged;
4. the veins and arteries which provide blood to the brain being torn.

The latter can lead to bleeding (haemorrhage) and lack of oxygen to the brain causing damage or death of nerve cells. As a result the messages that are sent through these damaged areas are disrupted. This type of damage is called 'primary damage'. There can also be 'secondary damage' if the head injury causes swelling in the brain, brain infection or not enough oxygen to get to the brain (hypoxia) because of breathing difficulties or very low blood pressure.

Often in a severe head injury the front of the brain (frontal lobes) and lower sides of the brain (temporal lobes) are the areas that receive the most damage. This is because there are sharp parts of the skull that stick out here and during a severe head injury the brain moves within the skull causing damage in these areas. There is also often damage to the nerve cell tails (axons) over lots of areas of the brain due to the brain stretching or rubbing against itself (diffuse axonal shearing).

Improvement after Head Injury

Even though there is no such thing as a 'typical' head injury, after very severe head injuries there is always *some degree* of natural healing of the brain. Generally most recovery takes place over the first one to two years. The improvements then tend to slow down and level out. Small amounts of natural recovery can continue for a long time afterwards, although these tend to be much smaller improvements compared with those that occur in the first year or two. Improvements in how a person copes with everyday life, however, can go on indefinitely as they learn to adapt and find ways around the difficulties that arise. It is impossible to say early on after a very severe head injury how much natural improvement is likely to occur and whether the person will get back to 99 per cent of their original mental capacity or 85 per cent or 50 per cent, etc. This becomes clearer as time goes on. Some permanent reduction in mental ability, however, is usual after a very severe head injury.

The natural recovery after severe head injury is not fully understood, but it probably involves:

1. the chemicals which transmit the electrical message in the brain cells (neurons) settling down and regaining some of their original efficiency;
2. some of the damaged neurons or their connections repairing themselves;
3. the swelling and bruising in the brain reducing, causing the neurons in these areas to function more efficiently.

It may possibly also involve undamaged areas of the brain taking on some of the responsibilities that damaged areas used to do (neuroplasticity). However, not everyone agrees about how much this can occur.

Cognitive Rehabilitation

As well as the natural recovery of the brain following a head injury, significant improvements in a person's day-to-day life can occur as a result of *cognitive rehabilitation*. Unfortunately there is very little evidence that 'brain training' exercises help recovery or strengthen cognitive skills after an injury. Generally speaking, the person will get better at the exercises but there will be little improvement in their day-to-day thinking skills. Cognitive rehabilitation therefore usually involves: providing detailed information about head injury to the person and their family or friends; assessing the person's thinking skills to identify their specific strengths and weaknesses; finding practical strategies to solve the problems that the brain injury causes, e.g. using a diary to help memory and planning problems. It often includes relearning specific skills a person needs for everyday life. This not only helps the person relearn the skills they need but may also help stimulate the areas of the brain responsible for these things, therefore aiding its natural recovery.

It can also include the process of adjusting to the changes that have occurred as a result of the injury. This often involves difficult emotions and is a slow process. Some people view it as a kind of emotional journey involving challenges along the way but with positive emotional growth occurring as understanding, insight and realistic hope are developed. For some this means accepting at least part of themselves as being a 'new person'. This means that while they are the same person as before, they learn to accept some different characteristics in their make-up.

Mild Traumatic Brain Injury and Post-concussion Symptoms

Definition

The term 'mild traumatic brain injury' (MTBI) often includes both mild and moderate injuries. When using the 'MTBI' abbreviation in this book it will mean both of these. The other common term for these injuries is 'mild head injury' (MHI) and clinicians often use either to mean exactly the same thing. Other common terms include 'concussion' and 'minor head injury'. They are usually defined as injuries resulting in:

1. unconsciousness of less than fifteen minutes;
2. post-traumatic amnesia of less than twenty-four hours;
3. an initial Glasgow Coma Scale score of 13–15;
4. no evidence of significant brain injury from basic neurological indicators (see below).

Brain Scans and Serious Complications after MTBI

Brain scans in the early phase after a head injury are undertaken to detect the presence of bleeding in the brain or other damage that might require neurosurgery or other medical treatments. In themselves they do not measure the severity of the injury. It is therefore rare for someone with a mild traumatic brain injury to require a brain scan, particularly if:

1. they have a high Glasgow Coma Scale score (i.e. they are conscious and are responsive in a conversation);
2. they have no obvious physical symptoms of a brain injury (e.g. weakness in one or both arms or legs);
3. there are no key early indicators of a potentially significant brain injury.

Unfortunately not having a brain scan can feel like the MTBI has not been fully assessed or that something significant 'might have been missed'.

Key Factors for Further Medical Assessment

Some of the key factors that indicate that further medical assessment is immediately required include: the pupils in the eyes not reacting normally when light is shone into them ('Pupils Equal and Reactive to Light' [PEARL]); losses or deteriorating levels of consciousness (e.g. severe drowsiness; inability to be woken; experiencing fits, faints or collapses); cerebrospinal fluid leaking from the ears or nose (this is a clear liquid that surrounds the brain and acts as a 'cushion' for it); persistent vomiting; increasing disorientation or confusion; difficulties understanding or producing coherent speech; deafness, tinnitus or bleeding from one or both ears; blurred or double vision; problems with balance or walking; weakness or numbness in one or both arms or legs; severe, worsening or persisting headaches that are not relieved by over-the-counter painkillers. These serious but rare complications usually occur within the first few hours, days or weeks after a mild traumatic brain injury (rather than months) and if experienced mean that the person should seek immediate medical assessment at a hospital Accident and Emergency (A&E) department.

Differences between Mild Traumatic Brain Injury and Severe Head Injury

In nearly all respects a MTBI is very different from a severe or very severe head injury.

First, there is usually no clear-cut evidence of any significant brain injury. Second, there is a full expectation of complete recovery over a relatively short period of time. Third, post-concussion symptoms are not symptoms that *only* occur after a head injury and they can be caused or made worse by a large range of non-head injury factors like stress, pain or low mood. Fourth, MTBI is much more common than severe head injury with a lifetime risk of 2–10 per cent – incredibly large numbers of people therefore experience one at some point in their lives.

Post-concussion Symptoms

Post-concussion symptoms (PCS) are a range of difficulties that often occur as a result of a mild traumatic brain injury. They include headaches, dizziness, fatigue, irritability, sleep disturbance, reduced day-to-day memory, poor concentration, taking longer to think, 'muzzy'-headedness, depression, anxiety, tinnitus, blurred or double vision, sensitivity to light or noise, frustration, nausea, restlessness and sensitivity to alcohol. For the vast majority these symptoms completely resolve over the first few weeks or months.

Case Study 1

Graham, a twenty-four year-old trainee solicitor, suffered a head injury as the result of a head-on car collision. When the ambulance arrived at the scene he was still unconscious and the paramedics assessed his Glasgow Coma Scale score as 5. He was taken to the nearest hospital with a neurosurgical department, placed in an induced coma for two weeks and treated in intensive care for this time. A CT brain scan showed small areas of contusion (bruising) in the frontal and temporal areas of the brain. After coming out of his coma he was still quite confused for a further four weeks. It was not until six or seven weeks after the accident that he consistently remembered what had happened to him, what the days and the dates were, and who had visited him the previous day and what they had spoken about. He could also not remember anything of the week before the accident. He had two months of in-patient rehabilitation and a further eighteen months of community rehabilitation.

His head injury was classed as 'very severe' and resulted in some permanent brain damage affecting his day-to-day memory, thinking speed, multi-tasking abilities and organizational skills. He also got tired much more easily and was more prone to irritability and being 'snappy'. Despite doing very well with his rehabilitation he eventually realized that he would not be able to complete his legal training because of his difficulties and successfully adjusted in the long-term to working twenty-three hours a week in a legal-support role for a large firm of solicitors.

Case Study 2

Susan, a forty-eight year-old administrator in an insurance company, suffered a head injury as the result of a horse-riding accident. Her friend who was riding with her thought she may have been knocked out for a few seconds but quickly 'came round' even though she was 'groggy' and confused. When the ambulance arrived her Glasgow Coma Scale score was assessed as being 14 as she was unable to describe what had happened to her or what the year, month or day were.

She was assessed at the local A&E department. No brain scan was required and by the time she left, three hours later, she was fully aware of what had happened to her and knew the day, month and year. Her head injury was classed as 'mild to moderate' and her partner was asked to keep a watchful eye on her for the first twenty-four hours as she was still feeling very tired, 'foggy' and had a severe headache. These symptoms slowly improved and she felt close to being fully recovered after two weeks signed off work. She then returned to work on a part-time basis doing three hours a day, three days a week. These hours were built up slowly and by six weeks she was back to full-time work and she felt '100 per cent her normal self'.

Managing Early Symptoms

In the early stages symptoms are normally caused by the subtle and temporary brain injury the person has sustained. During the first few days or weeks of having post-concussion symptoms, the best advice is not to return to work or to normal levels of activity too quickly and initially to plan a fairly light schedule of activities that can be very slowly increased in a paced and systematic manner over time. Performing routine and non-stressful tasks and avoiding too many activities that put the person under pressure can help this pacing process. Stress can aggravate PCS so minimizing tasks requiring a lot of cognitive speed, effort or concentration can also be of benefit. When people are more sensitive to the effects of alcohol as a result of their injury it is normally best that they abstain from it for an initial period. It should then be slowly reintroduced with very gradual increases while continuing to monitor the effects. Returning to work or normal activities should also be done in a slow-paced and structured way. Stress can aggravate post-concussion symptoms and can easily cause a vicious cycle to develop. This occurs when PCS causes stress, which in turn leads to more PCS and so on. This is summarized in the diagram below:

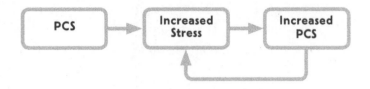

Keeping an Eye on Your Life Demands

One of the most helpful ways to stop these cycles developing is to keep a watchful eye on the day-to-day demands that you are taking on. If your life demands are kept even slightly lower than your available mental resources then you are likely to prevent the cycle. If post-concussion symptoms do get worse it often means that your life demands have very slowly increased over time without being noticed and have started to exceed your resources. This can often happen when you start to return to work or normal activities as the stress levels can be significantly higher than when just recuperating. Noticing increasing fatigue or irritability, or the worsening of other PCS, can therefore be a helpful warning sign that demands are getting too large and need to be reduced. Without this adjustment the stress and worry of deteriorating symptoms can quickly place even greater cognitive and emotional demands on you and you can feel even less in control of your life and able to manage your daily tasks. Further vicious cycles can therefore quickly develop in this way also. The following diagrams summarize how demands and resources can be balanced effectively:

Before the Injury – Resources are Greater than the Demands, Resulting in No Stress

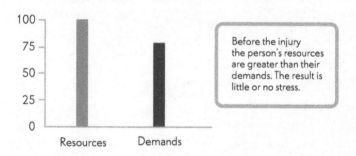

Before the injury the person's resources are greater than their demands. The result is little or no stress.

After the Injury – Resources are Reduced But the Demands Remain the Same
(The Result is Increased Stress and PCS)

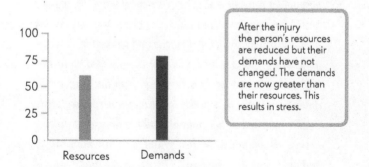

After the injury the person's resources are reduced but their demands have not changed. The demands are now greater than their resources. This results in stress.

After the Injury – Reducing the Demands Leads to Reduced Stress

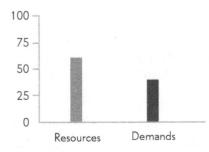

The person reduces their demands so that their resources are once again greater than their demands. The result is little or no stress.

Case Study

Menaz, a thirty-four year-old mother of three and part-time book-keeper, suffered a mild traumatic brain injury and whiplash injury as the result of a rear-end car shunt. She was seen briefly in Accident and Emergency, did not require a brain scan and was discharged with a Mild Head Injury leaflet. This listed a range of symptoms to look out for and if experienced meant that she should return to the hospital for reassessment. She experienced a number of post-concussion symptoms including tiredness, poor day-to-day memory, irritability, mental fatigue and reduced multi-tasking abilities. She also had a lot of neck and head pain. Her husband took two weeks off work to help her manage the children and after three weeks she felt completely recovered.

She returned to her normal working hours but quickly noticed deterioration in her symptoms and more angry outbursts with her children. This, unsurprisingly, caused her to think that there was something seriously wrong with her brain and that this had been missed in A&E. Over the following few weeks more deterioration occurred and she eventually saw her general practitioner as by now she was really worried about what was happening to her. He explained that the first worsening of her symptoms was caused by the increased demands of returning to work. This resulted in worries and stress, which themselves became extra demands on her, causing further vicious cycles to develop. This explanation helped calm her concerns and lower her stress. She reduced her working hours down to a minimum and built them up slowly over the next two months. At this point she was back to full-time hours and she and husband felt she had made a full recovery.

Persisting Symptoms

Unfortunately a very small minority of patients suffer from persisting or long-term post-concussion symptoms. In a few cases some PCS can be permanent. This will often mean that the term 'mild traumatic brain injury' does not in any way adequately describe the consequences of the injury. Ongoing PCS can be very disabling indeed and affect almost all aspects of life. Such difficulties are frequently called a 'hidden disability' or an 'invisible disability' as the person usually looks fine and in a range of situations may show no obvious effects of the injury. Persisting PCS are often labelled as the 'post-concussion syndrome' but not everyone agrees that the term 'syndrome' is a helpful way of thinking about these symptoms. Stress, worry, anxiety, irritability and low mood can also develop as a response to the large increases in the effort needed to try to cope with PCS. This is called the 'Coping Hypothesis' theory of mild traumatic brain injury.

Other Factors that Can Cause the Same Symptoms

Post-concussion-type symptoms are not very specific and nearly all of them can be caused by things completely unrelated to a MTBI. These include: chronic pain, stress, low mood, reduced quality or quantity of sleep, the emotional consequences of a psychological trauma (post-traumatic stress), physical or cognitive symptoms caused by emotional disturbances (somatoform problems), anxiety and chronic fatigue problems. Indeed, quite a number of normal, healthy adults will report some of these problems in their everyday life without any of these factors. Unfortunately the circumstances that cause a MTBI (e.g. road traffic accidents, assaults, serious accidents, bomb blasts in conflict situations, etc.) can also cause these other factors to be present. These might include: pain from physical injuries; post-traumatic stress; difficulty getting one's life back to normal; stress arising from a compensation claim (if someone else caused the injury); feeling more vulnerable or 'shook up'.

Post-Traumatic Stress

Post-traumatic stress (PTS) is a deep emotional response to an intensely traumatic experience. When these symptoms are very severe they are sometimes termed post-traumatic stress disorder (PTSD). They result in the person re-experiencing many of the painful feelings and memories that occurred at the time of the trauma. These can take the form of nightmares, flashbacks, intrusive memories or images, feeling like the person is reliving the event or distressing feelings when things bring the event to mind. Sometimes these are particularly powerful or more frequent when first waking up or when intoxicated. The painful feelings can cause people to actively avoid things that remind them of the event and to avoid thinking or talking about it altogether.

Many clinicians used to think that all head injuries offered complete protection against post-traumatic stress disorders (PTSD) as the amnesia caused by the head injury would stop the person having any memories of the event and therefore make them unable to re-experience recollections of it in any way. Recent research, however, shows that this is only true after severe head injuries where the likelihood of developing PTSD is low (possibly 5 per cent or less). The research shows that it is not true after mild traumatic brain injury and that these injuries offer no protection. In fact, some clinicians believe that they may actually slightly increase the chances of experiencing the disorder. This is because the processing and storing of information at the time of the event may be disrupted by the head injury or cause difficulties later on when trying to piece memories together coherently. This might therefore make the recovery from the emotional trauma more difficult. After events like road traffic accidents, the likelihood of developing PTSD has been found to be about the same whether a MTBI is experienced or not (10–25 per cent).

There are four main situations where post-traumatic stress disorder and mild traumatic brain injury occur together:

1. where post-traumatic amnesia (PTA, i.e. amnesia caused by the head injury) is absent or short so there are lots of memories of the event;
2. where there is a traumatic 'island of memory' during PTA. This is a very brief, isolated memory within the period of PTA when everything else is not remembered;
3. where there is a fear response that occurs outside of conscious awareness such that reminders of the event automatically trigger extremely strong emotional reactions (usually fear) despite there being no conscious memory of it whatsoever – like an emotional reflex reaction;
4. where the person has images or 'pseudo-memories' of the event from what they know or presume to know about it (e.g. from photos relating to it, eyewitness accounts of it, etc.).

'Windows' of Vulnerability

When post-concussion symptoms do persist for more than a few months it is likely that some of these other factors will in some way start to play a role, e.g. the natural and normal worry of not having achieved a full recovery. The table below shows how just some of the non-brain injury factors may play a part at different times after a MTBI if someone has persisting symptoms. This is called the 'Windows of Vulnerability' theory of PCS:

Time after injury	Possible emerging factors
0–24 hours (immediate symptoms)	Mainly temporary brain injury factors.
1 day–4 weeks (early symptoms)	Overdoing and failing tasks. Increase in life demands following recuperation. Thinking symptoms are caused by serious medical conditions that have been missed. Difficulties coping with cognitive impairments. Initial concerns regarding the length of time for symptoms/disabilities to resolve. Stress and frustration regarding the 'mild' severity of the head injury compared to the severity of symptoms/disabilities.
1–6 months (medium-term symptoms)	Unhelpful pre-injury coping responses for managing abnormal life events. Inability to complete tasks. Frustration and 'mind over matter' coping not working. Concerns regarding potential permanence of symptoms. Unhelpful strategies for coping with uncertainty (particularly the uncertain cause(s) of symptoms). Misperception of having suffered a severe brain injury.
Over 6 months (long-term or possibly permanent symptoms)	Lack of understanding/belief from others. Compensation-claim factors. Issues relating to adjusting to long-term disability. Unhelpful 'secondary' coping strategies (those used when initial strategies do not work).

Source: N. S. King, 'Post-concussion syndrome: clarity amid the controversy?', *British Journal of Psychiatry*, 183 (2003), 276–8. Reprinted with permission.

Different Opinions

Unfortunately, when post-concussion symptoms persist there are often very differing opinions from clinicians about what causes them to be prolonged and how best they can be helped. There are five main reasons for this complication:

1. the uncertainty about the cause of long-term PCS (whether they are due to a subtle brain injury or other factors or both);
2. the fact that there is a very large range of outcomes after apparently identical injuries (from no symptoms at all to very disabling and permanent PCS);
3. the fact that most people get completely better and quite quickly;
4. a lack of hard evidence of a significant brain injury being present even when there are very significant long-term disabilities;
5. the fact that some PCS are very rare after more severe head injuries e.g. sensitivity to light, nausea, headaches.

Non-Head Injury Factors

Some clinicians think that in the early stages PCS are caused by a subtle but completely reversible brain injury, and that long-term post-concussion-type symptoms are always due to non-head injury factors. They might be aware that mild traumatic brain injury can cause subtle brain damage, which shows up on the newer, more sensitive brain scanners that are normally only used in research centres. However, they would argue that this damage is only present for some people and that even when there is damage to be seen it often completely resolves within the first few months. Also, even if the damage is still present years later it would be too slight to cause any difficulties for a patient. They might also point to the studies that show that: stress makes PCS worse; psychological factors often best indicate who might go on to suffer long-term PCS; symptoms can worsen when patients develop expectations of what symptoms they are likely to experience, which then become 'over-focused' on and therefore noticed more and more; many people with prolonged symptoms also have other difficulties they have to deal with, which could cause PCS-type problems, e.g. pain, post-traumatic stress or other life stresses. In other words, the symptoms may not change as time goes on but the causes of them do.

Subtle Brain Injury

Other clinicians believe that persisting post-concussion symptoms are always caused by the mild brain injury itself. They might point to evidence from the studies that have used the more sensitive brain scanners or they may have seen a lot of patients who have no 'other factors' but who still have long-term PCS. Some clinicians may just be unaware of the other factors that cause the same difficulties, e.g. stress causing day-to-day memory problems, pain causing poor concentration problems, anxiety causing blurred vision, etc.

Both Subtle Brain Injury and 'Other' Factors

Still others will be open to the possibility that both head injury and non-head injury factors, and the interactions between them, can be responsible for prolonged symptoms.

Unfortunately this means that the person with the MTBI may get very different, and sometimes opposite, opinions about PCS depending on which clinicians they see. Indeed, there is some evidence that the opinion a patient may get on their persisting PCS will be influenced by the type of clinician they see. In one study neurosurgeons had a tendency to favour non-head injury explanations of symptoms whilst neuropsychologists tended to favour subtle brain injury ones! Clearly this can be extremely unsettling, frustrating and confusing, and can add to the uncertainty and stress already present.

Brain Injury vs Non-Brain Injury Factors

If clinicians discuss non-brain injury factors with you it can easily feel like they are suggesting that your problems are 'not real' or are 'all in your mind'. This should definitely not be the case as your difficulties are just as real and disabling regardless of whether brain injury, non-brain injury or both factors are the cause. The fact that emotional and psychological factors can cause physical symptoms, or problems with certain kinds of thinking skills, does not mean that the difficulties are any less real or severe than if they are caused by a brain injury.

Emotional factors can play a part even if you do not feel particularly stressed or depressed. Physical difficulties or problems with thinking skills caused by emotional factors can sometimes act as a kind of protection or 'shield' from feelings that you are not aware of and which are not ready to be fully experienced by you. These are sometimes called 'somato-form' problems. This can make it even harder to judge how much brain-injury or non-brain injury factors are involved. Indeed, sometimes the only way to really make this judgement is to fully address all the treatable non-brain injury ones and assume that if there are any post-concussion symptoms left after this they might be due to brain-injury factors. In many ways the more your difficulties are actually caused by non-brain injury factors the better it is – as these are the ones that have the best chance of being fully overcome.

Vicious Cycles

Whilst there are differing opinions from clinicians about the persisting difficulties experienced after a mild traumatic brain injury there are a number of facts that are known about long-term PCS:

1. We know that age (possibly with a broad cut off of being over forty) and gender (being female) can increase the likelihood of experiencing prolonged post-concussion-type symptoms.
2. We know that a large number of people with per-sisting symptoms may have factors over and above their traumatic brain injury to manage, which might contribute to their difficulties e.g. post-traumatic stress reactions, ongoing pain, physical limitations

due to orthopaedic injuries, pre-injury or post-injury stressors in their lives.

3. We know that any direct effects of a mild brain injury will improve over time – the natural healing processes that occur in the brain, however, can be very slow, e.g. after very severe brain injuries maximum improvement may take up to two years.

4. We know that any brain injury factors will reduce over time and non-head injury factors may well increase – especially if the person struggles to understand and manage their PCS. This is demonstrated in the graph below.

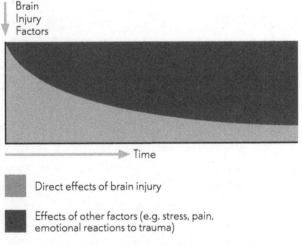

Brain Injury Factors

Time

■ Direct effects of brain injury

■ Effects of other factors (e.g. stress, pain, emotional reactions to trauma)

Source: S. Potter and R. G. Brown, 'CBT and persisting PCS: integrating conceptual issues and practical aspects of treatment', *Neuropsychological Rehabilitation*, 22:1 (2012), 1–25 (after W. A. Lishman, 'Physiogenesis and psychogenesis in the "post-concussion syndrome"', *British Journal of Psychiatry*, 153 [1988], 460–9). Reprinted with permission.

5. We know that, regardless of the causes of the different symptoms, they can become mutually exacerbating so that many vicious cycles between them develop as time goes on, e.g. reduced concentration causing increased stress, causing further concentration difficulties, causing more stress, etc. Natural personality characteristics like perfectionism, 'all-or-nothing' approaches to dealing with problems or a strong desire to control things may then cause additional vicious cycles.

Case Study

Jenny, a twenty-nine year-old hairdresser, describes herself as 'always being a bit of a perfectionist' and a 'control freak' with very high standards for herself. She is a person who has overcome many challenges in her life – mainly by working harder and harder and subscribing to the philosophy of 'no pain, no gain'. She is very successful with her own salon, she is a high achiever in most things and generally she commits herself wholeheartedly to anything she takes on in her life. She sustained a mild traumatic brain injury as a result of a pedestrian road-traffic accident.

For the first four weeks she suffered with severe headaches, tiredness, reduced concentration and taking longer to think. She was unable to return to work and strongly felt that she was letting her stylists and her clients down. She also felt 'like a fraud' for being off work, particularly as she had been told in Accident and Emergency that she would be 'fully recovered in one to two weeks'.

43

She was '80 per cent her normal self' when she forced herself to return to the salon one month after the accident. However, she found that she could not deal with all of her clients, made a lot of mistakes in her cutting, struggled with her accounting and was 'snappy' with her staff. This resulted in strong feelings of being a failure, guilt and anxiety, which made her focus her attention more and more on the mistakes she made rather than on her successes. She forced herself to try to work long, hard hours on 'good days', only to find that she had two or three 'bad days' afterwards where she could not work at all. She described these as 'payback days'. This 'boom-bust' approach made her feel less and less in control of her life. All of these factors added to her mental load and by six months she felt no better than in the early days after it.

She was eventually referred to a clinical neuropsychologist. After a discussion about the factors causing her problems, some brief cognitive behavioural therapy was undertaken looking at Jenny's perfectionism. She discovered that while it protected her from some underlying low self-esteem it had only added to her problems since her injury. Some pacing and fatigue management strategies were put into place and Jenny 'gave herself permission' to reduce her working hours so that she could regain some feeling of control in her life. By eighteen months after the MTBI she had slowly returned to full-time hours and felt fully recovered – so much so that she only very rarely thought about the accident.

An Example of a Vicious Cycle

An example of just one common vicious cycle is below. It shows how someone going to a party might worry about not being able to remember people's names. This is seen as a 'memory challenge', which leads to unhelpful thoughts and increased stress. These in turn lead to further problems, making their memory worse and worse:

**Vicious Cycle –
Worry About Remembering Someone's Name**

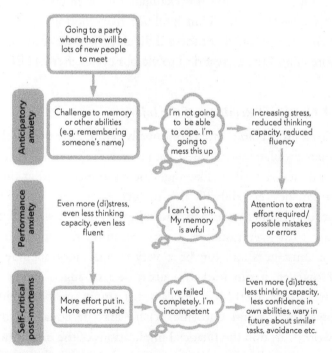

Source: Adapted from S. Potter and R. G. Brown, 'CBT and persisting PCS: integrating conceptual issues and practical aspects of treatment', *Neuropsychological Rehabilitation*, 22:1 (2012), 1–25. Reprinted with permission.

Legal Proceedings

For some, being involved in legal proceedings because of their mild traumatic brain injury can be a very specific form of stress that powerfully contributes to vicious cycles. Such proceedings are common if your MTBI was caused by somebody else. They could involve a compensation claim against whoever was responsible or a criminal case against them. Unfortunately these can take a long time to complete and cause substantial additional stress while they are ongoing. Compensation claims, for example, can often take at least a few years to resolve. Unhelpful negative emotions caused by being in the middle of these difficult procedures can therefore contribute a great deal to vicious cycles after MTBI.

A Continual Reminder of the Injury

Legal proceedings often continually remind the person that their problems were due to someone else's fault. This can easily foster feelings like anger or resentment and at times it can be very difficult not to 'get stuck' with emotions around blame, unfairness and injustice. The desire for the law to deliver justice is a very common feeling in these circumstances and can be a very strong emotion indeed. However, it can lead to a great deal of anger, worry or stress, particularly if it appears that things are proceeding away from a just outcome. There may be equally strong worries around the financial implications of the case. These too can easily dominate your thoughts and feelings even when proceedings are going through a lull.

Feelings Being 'Churned Up'

If there is post-traumatic stress or other strong emotions associated with the circumstances of the MTBI it can often feel like these are continually being 'churned up' by the proceedings. You may feel that you are being forced to constantly relive the event but in such a way that makes you only feel worse rather than better. It can sometimes feel like you are being re-traumatised each time you have to go through the event.

It is not unusual for you to have to see a number of medical experts, in addition to your legal representatives, as part of the proceedings. This too can feel like things are being 'churned up'. It also can mean that you receive very different opinions about your problems as there can be even more controversy and debate about the nature of post-concussion symptoms in legal settings than in clinical ones. Unsurprisingly, very different but confidently expressed expert opinions can cause confusion and worry in themselves. It is also not unusual for a person in the middle of legal proceedings to sometimes feel like they are being accused of lying, 'swinging the lead' or exaggerating things. You can at times feel like you are not the victim in the process but the one who is on trial!

Other Stresses

Other stress can arise because, in a strange way, what may be good for your legal proceedings may at times be bad for your real-life progress and vice versa. For example, it may be better legally if your symptoms don't get better, are more severe and you don't manage to reclaim important parts of normality back, e.g. by slowly returning to work. On the other hand, these might be exactly the things you are working on, possibly with a clinician's help in order to overcome your PCS.

Further stress can arise when, at certain times, there are many appointments to attend, important reports to read or meetings to take part in. Playing your part in these procedures can sometimes feel like a full-time job in itself. On top of all this almost everyone dreads the thought of having to go to court and giving evidence (even though the vast majority of compensation claims are settled without having to go).

It is hardly surprising that with such a wide range of possible stresses surrounding legal proceedings some people feel that they cannot fully 'move on' with their problems until their 'legal chapter' is fully closed by the case coming to an end. If the legal outcome, however, is not ultimately a good one and it feels like justice has not been done, anger and other very strong feelings can continue even after the case has finished. The negative impact of legal procedures can therefore be substantial. Many people, though, find the completion of their case a very positive step in their progress and feel that when this chapter closes they are able to 'move on' in quite a powerful way.

What Helps?

Get the Right Kind of Solicitor

If you are involved in a compensation claim one of the most important things in helping you manage the stress around the legal proceedings is to make sure that your solicitor is a specialist in the area of personal injury claims and head injury, and has good experience of mild traumatic brain injury cases. Because MTBI and post-concussion symptoms can be particularly controversial and confusing in the legal field it is very important that you have high levels of confidence in your legal representatives. A good solicitor will not in any way be offended by you asking about their experience of MTBI or how many cases they have undertaken previously in this area. You do also have the right to change your solicitor after the process has started, so this is always an option if you have misgivings. Local and national head-injury self-help groups will often have lists of legal specialists they recommend and they can be a good place to start if you are unsure where to look.

Keep Your 'Legal-life' Separate from Real Life

The second most important thing in managing legal procedures is to try and create as much emotional distance as you can from the things required for the legal process and your 'real life'. Your real-life progress is the most important thing to stay focused on and the more you can separate this from your 'legal life' the better. If you can picture your 'legal life' as something to be placed in a 'bubble' you may be able, in your mind, to 'put it on a high shelf' out of the way to help with this separation. You will have to take the bubble down from time to time to deal with your 'legal life', but you can then replace it on the shelf, out of the way, until needed again. This will help to make sure that the legal proceedings work around your real life as much as possible rather than the other way round.

Use Cognitive Behavioural Strategies

Inevitably there will be times when the proceedings will be stressful. Acknowledging these feelings and implementing some of the strategies in the 'Anxiety and Stress' part of Section 2 of this book will further help you manage things, e.g. by recognizing and challenging unhelpful thoughts associated with the legal case.

Shaken Sense of Self Identity

People who experience prolonged PCS can often have a shaken sense of their own identity as they are unable to do many of the things they used to do and their roles within work, family, with their partner or socially can be jeopardized or dramatically changed. If this occurs at the same time that they are struggling to understand what is happening to them, then broader unconscious perceptions can be questioned. This can be particularly difficult if they include assumptions about how stable, reliable and predictable the world and the person are. Cycles of fear, failure, avoidance, anxiety, low self-esteem, reduced confidence and feelings of alienation can consequently easily develop. This can be especially so if the person previously relied on high levels of achievement or perfectionism to maintain a feeling of self-worth or if they were used to high levels of control in their lives.

What Helps?

Listing Your Symptoms and All the Factors that Could Be Involved

A very useful first step in helping someone suffering from prolonged post-concussion-type symptoms is to make a list of all the problems they currently experience. The second step is then to make a list of all the head-injury and non-head-injury factors that might possibly be contributing to the symptoms. The third step is then to decide which symptoms could be causing vicious cycles of problems as there are often many of these with prolonged post-concussion symptoms. The fourth step is then to explore how the difficulties may have affected the way the person feels, thinks or behaves and any vicious cycles that may have developed in these areas.

Having Help in this Process

It is vitally important that you do not worry if you find it difficult to do this on your own as it can be very difficult indeed to be able to recognize all the possible factors that might be relevant without professional help. Indeed, a clinician's first role is often to help you to see the 'wood from the trees' in this process. It is very common for someone with persisting PCS to need the help of a clinician.

This may be especially important if it is difficult to stand back from the problems; if it is difficult to know where to start because things seem overwhelming; or if some of the solutions seem to 'oppose each other'. 'Opposing strategies' might arise, for example, when using a diary to help you with your memory difficulties. This strategy may be very effective for remembering things but causes you to never get the chance to test out whether your memory without a 'back-up' is in fact better than you think it is, e.g. because you have become more and more focused on 'normal' memory lapses over time and this has exaggerated 'memory problems' in your mind. The diary strategy may also not allow you to challenge negative thoughts about how bad it will be if you do experience 'memory failures'. In these situations it may be particularly useful for a clinician to work through these 'opposing' strategies with you.

A clinical neuropsychologist will often be the clinician best able to help you with this process but this will not always be the case. Unfortunately, the wrong kind of help can sometimes make things seem worse as it may lead to an inaccurate understanding of the problems and 'burden' you with self-blame and reduced hope. If you have not found the right kind of help you may need to be persistent in looking for it as it is not always easy to find. At times a less specialist clinician with the help of this book may be more effective for you than an expert one with fixed and rigid ideas about your difficulties.

Box Diagram

Sometimes your clinician will summarize all the different factors in a box diagram to create an individualized explanation of the specific difficulties and their causes. One 'box' can be tackled at a time and vicious cycles can be reduced and 'virtuous cycles' increased. By slowing tackling the difficulties 'one box at a time' substantial improvements can be made in both reducing PCS and effectively managing any that remain. The good news is that there are many scientifically proven ways of tackling the individual 'boxes', e.g. stress may be helped by stress-management training taken from mental health resources; day-to-day memory problems may be helped by cognitive rehabilitation strategies taken from severe brain-injury resources; unhelpful feelings/thoughts/behaviour may be helped by specific forms of psychological interventions such as cognitive behavioural therapy. There is therefore nearly always optimism for improvement with the right professional help.

Case Study

Simon, a forty-six year-old teacher, suffered a MTBI as the result of a road-traffic accident caused by someone else. After eighteen months he was still experiencing a large number of very problematic symptoms that seemed to be getting worse over time. He had not been able to return to work and was becoming more and more concerned about his difficulties. In particular, he could not understand how such major disabilities could result from an accident

53

that had been described by the police as 'minor' and a head injury that was described by clinicians as 'mild'. As well as suffering a MTBI he had ongoing pain from the whiplash injury he experienced and post-traumatic stress symptoms due to the terrifying nature of the crash. In addition, he was pursuing a compensation claim against the driver who caused the accident. His quite complicated 'box diagram' was as follows:

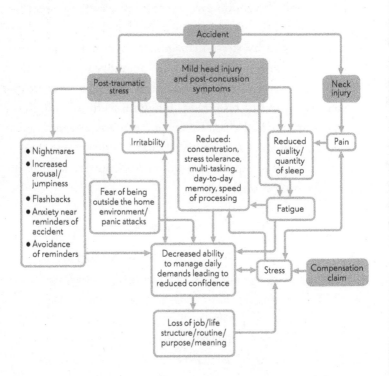

With the help of his clinical neuropsychologist he was quickly able to identify which 'boxes' he wanted to tackle first and improvements were steadily made in most areas, changing the vicious cycles to virtuous ones. One of the key turning points for Simon was creating some 'emotional distance' from his 'real life' and all that was going on with his compensation claim. He found that it 'kept on churning up' issues around the accident and caused him continually to question his understanding of his difficulties and how best to help them. He eventually was able to mentally put all his medicolegal proceedings 'into a bubble' and 'kept the bubble on a shelf'. He then only took the 'bubble' down to look at when the legal process required it but placed it back on the shelf straightaway afterwards. He found this stopped 'the legal things from "infecting" real-life'. He was eventually able to return to the classroom in a very graduated way, building up his hours slowly over time, and ultimately got back to full-time teaching even though one or two of his post-traumatic stress symptoms remained.

The Individualized Explanation

It is vitally important that any individualized explanation like the one above *is talked through and agreed upon* before starting treatment. Sometimes this needs a bit of discussion and refinement to find an understanding that 'fits' for both the person and their clinician. Once it has been established, though, it means that treatment can be focused on one factor at a time, depending on what is the highest priority for the person.

Different Ways of Helping

Once a shared understanding is established, a clinician might work with the person in a number of areas:

1. Helping to re-establish a shaken sense of self-identity by setting small goals to achieve or challenges to overcome.
2. Rebuilding external support systems and internal coping skills.
3. Helping those close to the person to understand the problems and how best they can support them.
4. Identifying factors that improve or worsen post-concussion symptoms, e.g. poor sleep leading to fatigue leading to concentration problems etc.
5. Minimizing 'boom-bust' oscillations between high and low levels of activity so that a stable base of sustainable-activity-level can be first established and then slowly and systematically increased.
6. Helping to gradually increase activity levels in terms of duration and/or intensity.
7. Exploring ways to *respond* differently to PCS rather than be stuck in the past (before the MTBI).
8. Examining ways in which thoughts relating to perfectionism, high achievement or being in complete

control of one's life might be replaced with more helpful ideas.

9. Exploring how increased effort and pushing oneself does not always result in increased achievement, i.e. that moderate levels of effort can lead to optimum achievement but that higher levels actually result in worse performance.

10. Exploring how consciously paying attention to the ways in which tasks are undertaken may lead to over-monitoring or 'over-thinking' and impede the more efficient 'autopilot' processes from working.

11. Examining how thoughts and ideas about failing tasks or anticipating failing tasks may impede performance.

Case Study 1

Hernandez, a thirty-six year-old Marine, suffered a mild traumatic brain injury as the result of a bomb blast whilst serving in Iraq. He described feeling 'quite shook up' for about four weeks afterwards and he experienced occasional nightmares about it, some irritability and was a bit more 'jumpy' and alert to danger during this time. He felt he made a 'pretty good recovery both emotionally and mentally' but was aware of some lingering changes in his ability to multi-task, concentrate for long periods of time and remember things in pressurized situations. He served out his time in Iraq and returned home. His problems improved but he did not feel that they ever entirely resolved.

Three months after returning home he was given a promotion. He quickly found himself struggling with the additional managerial and organizational responsibilities that his new post demanded. He had particular difficulties in reading and remembering new policies and in chairing long meetings. He worked longer and longer hours to keep on top of his paperwork. Despite this he still felt that he was not managing and secretly worried that his career had 'hit the blocks'. After nine months of 'hanging on by his fingernails' he was referred to the military's Brain Injury Team who assessed his problems thoroughly.

It was unclear to both Hernandez and the team whether he was suffering from subtle but permanent post-concussion symptoms that had been made worse by his increased responsibilities or whether his new role would always have been too big a step for his capabilities (he had always seen himself as 'never being very academic'). This may have resulted in him over-focusing more and more on 'normal' memory and concentration lapses, which everyone suffers from but usually ignore. A neuropsychological assessment revealed some mild difficulties with new learning and holding and manipulating information in his mind at the same time. These could, however, have been equally caused by stress or post-concussion symptoms, or both.

Hernandez put into place a number of strategies to help him manage his cognitive difficulties and eventually was able to 'job share' his role with another member of staff and to secure some additional administrative support. With his much lower job demands he eventually felt on top of his work and his worries and stress disappeared. At a follow-up appointment with the team three years after his injury he reported that he was managing well with the help of his strategies and that he was very happy with his life. He still, however, noticed residual memory and concentration differences compared to before the bomb blast, which he had accepted and around which he had successfully adapted some aspects of his life. It was therefore concluded that he had been left with some permanent PCS as the result of his MTBI as there were no other factors to account for his ongoing symptoms.

Case Study 2

Marie, a fifty-four-year-old nurse, sustained a MTBI after slipping on a floor at work and hitting her head. Eight years prior to this she had experienced a year-long period of depression following the break-up of her marriage and some difficulties at work with her manager. She was prescribed antidepressant medication during this time and received a short period of cognitive behavioural counselling, both of which she found helpful. With this support she managed to keep working and on top of her family responsibilities.

Following her MTBI she had severe problems with tiredness, poor concentration, reduced multi-tasking *abilities, sleep disturbance and sensitivity to noise. She was unable to return to work because of these problems and after six weeks was starting to feel low and anxious – particularly about letting her colleagues down and not being able to fulfil the high standards she had for herself. By six months she felt that she would never be able to return to the busy and high-pressured hospital environment and she became quite depressed. She was eventually assessed by a neurologist. She explained that Marie had initially experienced some severe post-concussion symptoms as a result of the MTBI. However, the depression and anxiety which then developed 'masked' the fact that her PCS had improved a great deal over time. The neurologist thought that her current symptoms were mainly caused by her emotional difficulties although they had originally been caused by the MTBI.*

She was referred to a cognitive behavioural therapist who identified that the high expectations she had of herself and her 'beating herself up' about not fulfilling her goals like she used to were key aspects of her thinking that maintained unhelpful vicious cycles. Treatment focused on helping Marie to become aware of a range of negative automatic thoughts and to challenge them. Relaxation training exercises were also introduced to help her manage the anxiety and stress that had built up. Marie herself realized that she needed to pace herself more and give herself breaks and rewards when tackling tasks. She implemented these strategies independently alongside taking up yoga.

She returned to her nursing role about a year after her accident on a part-time basis but found her responsibilities stressful rather than enjoyable and by eighteen months decided to take early retirement from her job. She became a part-time occupational health consultant for a large supermarket chain. In this role she had much more control over her working hours and her work practices. She started to enjoy her work-life again. Two-and-a-half years after the accident she was still enjoying this job although she was aware that she still did not sleep as well as before, that she got tired more easily and that she had to put in more effort when multi-tasking. At a follow-up appointment neither she nor her neurologist could be sure whether her residual difficulties were due to permanent PCS or her ongoing susceptibility to poor sleep and stress, or both. She had accepted these changes, however, and successfully adapted her life around them.

Overcoming Mild Traumatic Brain Injury

Section 2 of this book explores some of the most common factors that operate in MTBI and the ways in which they can be helped. It covers three areas of difficulties: thinking (cognitive), emotional and physical problems. Although these are treated separately it will be clear that there are huge interactions and overlaps between all of them. After applying the treatments most useful to you, you may completely overcome your post–concussion symptoms and eventually get back to 100 per cent normality. You may find, however, that some residual difficulties remain. Accepting these persisting problems, acknowledging that some things will not be the same as before and adapting to them can then become an important part of overcoming your PCS to the greatest possible degree.

SECTION 2

Thinking Difficulties

After a mild traumatic brain injury, the most common thinking (cognitive) difficulties are reduced thinking stamina (speed of information processing, mental speed or multi-tasking abilities) and day-to-day memory problems ('short-term memory' or remembering things since the injury). Occasionally some also report executive impairments (the ability to plan and coordinate goal-directed behaviour, think flexibly, have awareness about one's problems or think in abstract and non-concrete ways). However, these are much less typical. Reduced thinking stamina and day-to-day memory problems are also very common in people who experience ongoing pain, low mood, stress, anxiety and long-lasting fatigue. Regardless of the cause of these problems the next section outlines how some of these difficulties can present themselves and the **cognitive rehabilitation** management strategies that can help them. It also highlights how the general principles of cognitive rehabilitation may help.

'Brain Training' vs 'External' Strategies

Unfortunately, the brain is not like a muscle that can be exercised to improve different parts of it. There is therefore very little evidence that 'brain-training' mental exercises are effective in developing better thinking abilities. The person will usually improve their performance on the 'brain-training' exercise itself but there is unlikely to be any benefit in real-life abilities. The most effective cognitive rehabilitation strategies are therefore almost always practical and 'external', like always using a diary to 'back-up' your memory. These do not aim to improve the thinking abilities themselves but to find different ways of getting around thinking problems.

Having said this, it is important to maintain a reasonable level of mental stimulation to support good mental health but without 'overdoing it', which can lead to fatigue, irritability, stress or depression. The main focus in cognitive rehabilitation therefore is to develop a detailed understanding of the person's individual strengths and weaknesses in their thinking skills and creatively find alternative practical ways of achieving the best day-to-day functioning.

The Keys to Successful Strategies

It should first be noted that the keys to employing any strategy effectively are:

1. understanding your own individual cognitive strengths and weaknesses;
2. identifying only one new strategy to try at any one

time and being certain that this is the one *you* want as *your* goal;

3. acknowledging that until a new strategy has become a habit, it can take some effort to keep going with it. Usually after 4–8 weeks of consistent practice it will become a routine part of your daily life. If you are able to 'attach' the new strategy to a habit or routine you already have in place this can make it easier to learn. When you are able to use it almost on 'auto-pilot' it will then be an effective technique.

The following sections are designed to be read on a 'pick and choose' basis depending on the specific areas that are relevant to the reader.

Thinking Stamina

Your thinking stamina can be reduced for many different reasons (e.g. post-concussion symptoms, stress, low mood, pain or brain injury). If this happens you may find that you cope with the demands of everyday life less well and you need to pace yourself more carefully in managing your work and daily activities.

A Possible Cause

Reduced thinking stamina can occur because the information processing capacity of the brain is lowered. This means that the person is less able to process *as much* information as before or *as quickly* as before. In other words, the brain is more easily overloaded.

Symptoms You May Notice

Slowness – as information has to be taken on board in smaller amounts.

Distractibility – as it takes more effort to continue concentrating on an activity.

Forgetfulness – as less information can be stored at any one time.

Fatigue – as the brain has to work harder to process information.

Irritability – as the mind is under more stress.

Common Problems

Things that can be difficult during this time are:

1. activities that require multi-tasking or long periods of concentration, e.g. cooking a meal from scratch, reading a book, listening to a lecture or writing a report;
2. activities where more than one person is talking, e.g. meetings or social occasions;
3. activities where a lot of people are around you, e.g. shopping, working in a shared office or having young children wanting attention;

4. non-routine tasks, e.g. entertaining visitors or visiting unfamiliar places;
5. working fast to meet a deadline.

What Helps?

Things which can help include:

1. rearranging working environments to minimize background noise, 'busyness', unexpected events, time pressures and distractions, e.g. radio, computer, mobile phone or television;
2. breaking activities down into small sections with lots of small breaks in between, i.e. pacing tasks more;
3. doing *routine and familiar* tasks when fatigue and concentration are 'at their worst', e.g. at the end of an afternoon or end of a week;
4. doing *new and unfamiliar* tasks when you are 'at your best', e.g. in the morning or at the beginning of a week;
5. always using a diary to plan the day, pace yourself and remind yourself of things you need to do, e.g. appointments;
6. cutting down on non-essential activity – this may involve learning to say 'No' to things more: do not feel guilty about this;
7. taking many small breaks *before* impairments become apparent rather than 'pushing on' until forced to take a break due to 'cognitive overload';
8. returning to pre-injury activities very gradually and systematically over time.

9. identifying specific times or specific types of activity where fatigue, irritability, anxiety or frustration occur and making appropriate changes in these areas;

10. allowing extra time for tasks where multi-tasking is required.

Memory

Similarly, there are many different reasons why someone may have problems with their memory (e.g. post-concussion symptoms, stress, low mood, pain, brain injury). These problems generally occur for 'short-term' or day-to-day memory because older memories are usually much better established. In other words, it is new information that is often harder to remember and learn.

The Remembering Process

The process of remembering involves three different stages:

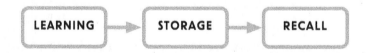

1. *Learning* – When you first concentrate on something.
2. *Storage* – The things you have learned are stored.
3. *Recall* – Getting information you have learnt to hand when you need it.

Memory is a bit like a filing cabinet where memories are

organized in an efficient filing system, making it easy to get information out when you want to remember it. There are many different files or types of memory: memory for faces, memory for events, memory for facts, memory for verbal information, memory for visual or spatial information, memory for physical acts and memory for the things we do on 'autopilot' because we have done them many times before. If any of these files are working less efficiently, memory lapses can occur i.e. the filing system is less effective or slowed down. Even if the information gets into the filing system and is stored, the system may be disorganized so the person gets muddled or confused. The memory can be affected because some of the files are less efficient at storing information (storage) or because the retrieval of information from the files is less efficient (recall).

Common Memory Problems

- Forgetting names, times, appointments, places, routes, phone numbers.

- Forgetting your train of thought, i.e. getting verbal blanks.

- Having words on the tip of your tongue and not being able to find the right words.

Things to Bear in Mind

1. Memory is not like a muscle and cannot be made better by doing exercises. Instead, it is better to adapt

69

to your changed memory and use strategies that can help overcome any difficulties, e.g. use a diary to write down appointments or write notes to remind you what you need to do.

2. Remember that nobody's memory is perfect. Therefore, try to avoid saying things like 'I'm stupid, I'm always forgetting things' as this may make you feel your memory is worse than it actually is.

3. Memory can be made worse by poor concentration so try not to do too many things at once. Your memory can also be affected by increases in anxiety, tiredness, irritability, frustration and stress, so try to keep these at manageable levels.

4. Try to be well organized in your everyday life, e.g. do certain things at certain times, have set routines and always leave things that you use a lot in their right place.

Helping Your Memory

The best way of helping difficulties with your memory is usually to accept the difficulties and adopt strategies to help get around the problems. It is then a matter of finding which strategy is most suited to your needs and lifestyle, and being disciplined about using it. At first, while you are getting used to a new strategy, you may find things get worse before they get better. This is normal and some perseverance is usually necessary for at least a few weeks.

Using a Diary, Electronic Reminders (e.g. Mobile Phone) or Notebook:

The most helpful memory strategy is often to use a diary, electronic reminder (e.g. mobile phone) or notebook in a very systematic way. It is most effective when used to plan and look ahead to things you need to do in the near future or to record important information you need to remember. The size and type of diary or reminder does not really matter but it is a good idea to get in the habit of carrying it around with you all the time in your pocket or handbag. This way you will always have it to hand when you need to write something down or check it. It is often a good idea to attach a pen or pencil to the diary or notebook so you always have something with which to write.

How to Use Your Diary, Electronic Reminder or Notebook:

Have a set time in the day when you write down your plans for the day or put in any future information in your diary, notebook, mobile phone etc. Generally, the best times are first thing in the morning or last thing at night. Try to get into the habit of checking your diary or device at regular intervals throughout the day, e.g. every hour or two.

What to Put in It:

Fill in the front pages with information such as names, phone numbers and addresses.

1. Every day put in appointments (e.g. doctor's appointments) including names, times, places and anything else you need to remember about the appointment (e.g. things you need to ask about).

2. Include things you need to know about the day (e.g. partner will be late in and where they are).
3. Include tasks that need to be done that day (e.g. pick cousin up from station).
4. Include things people have told you or you need to tell them (e.g. ask neighbour to return lawnmower).

As you complete tasks it is a good idea to cross them out or tick them off.

Other Memory Strategies

Other memory aids which can help are:

1. being as organized as possible in your everyday life, e.g. doing certain things at set times and having set routines;
2. writing down information on sticky notes and sticking them in places where you will need to remember the information;
3. using alarms on watches, mobile phones or clocks to remind you to do things like take medication or look at your diary/reminder;
4. using a mobile phone, computer or electronic organizer and setting reminders that prompt you to do things;
5. using a tape recorder/Dictaphone to help you remember things (e.g. when attending a meeting/ lecture);

6. asking a friend or relative to remind you to do things;
7. using a white board, notice board or calendar to quickly and regularly remind you of information (e.g. to buy someone's birthday present);
8. using satnav devices to find your way to new or unfamiliar places;
9. developing a tidy living and working environment where belongings are kept in the same, intuitively obvious, places and can easily be found; this helps to minimize demand on memory and problem-solving skills and make maximum use of non-conscious memory capacity;
10. taking pictures on a mobile phone as a reminder of significant things done previously in the day/week/ month, etc.;
11. systematically using written or photo journals for epi-sodic memory deficits (memory for personal events).
12. systematizing storage of household items with explicit labelling (e.g. colour coding);
13. using 'errorless learning' when learning new skills to minimize the need to 'unlearn' mistakes, i.e. getting others to prompt and cue you in such a way that no errors are made during a training process.

Mental Strategies

Some people also find mental memory strategies helpful. It should be noted that the degree of mental effort required for such 'internal' memory strategies often exceeds their usefulness for people with memory impairments. They can be useful, however, for specific tasks like remembering names of people or studying for an exam where external strategies are inappropriate. These are some of the most effective ones:

1. Repetition can help you to remember. Going over the information in your mind regularly can reinforce and help the learning stage of the memory process. You might also ask people to repeat information to help you remember what they have said.
2. Associations can help when you need to remember specific information, e.g. to remember the name Bob Fish, you might think of a person bobbing up and down with a fish on their head.
3. Chunking information together can help reduce the memory load, e.g. to remember a telephone number such as 01799486358, chunk the numbers together: 01-799-48-63-58.
4. Either visualizing or verbalizing what you have to remember can help, e.g. when trying to find your way in an unfamiliar place visualize landmarks to help you on your way back, or when remembering a route from a map, talk through instructions of how to get to your destination.

Executive Functioning

In a company the executive or boss has an important job. The executive has to: keep check on how the company is doing; plan for the future; put into practice different ways of working; and change how the company does things when circumstances change. The executive often has to stand back from the company and be flexible and creative.

The 'executive functioning' of the brain does a similar job to the boss in a company. Problems in this area of thinking can affect nearly all aspects of thinking and acting, and can show up in many different ways. The most common ways are:

1. *Coming up with ideas or intentions*
   People can find it difficult to think of things they would like to do. They can appear to have little energy, be less motivated or to have lost their 'get up and go'. Sometimes it seems like their 'spark' has gone. These problems can be mistaken for laziness or apathy.

2. *Starting and stopping movements or ideas*
   Moving parts of the body in particular ways may be difficult to get started. Sometimes movements can be more difficult to stop once they have got going. This can also happen when speaking or thinking. People can have problems in coming up with words and ideas or putting ideas into action. Once started, these may then be repeated when they would usually have stopped. This difficulty in stopping movements, words or thoughts is called 'perseveration'.

3. *Concrete thinking*
   People may find it difficult to be flexible with thoughts

or ideas. They can appear rigid or unable to 'let go' of fixed ideas. They can find it difficult to think in general or abstract ways, and can have problems in understanding jokes and irony or in answering open-ended questions, e.g. 'What would you like to do today?' Problems in putting themselves in the other person's shoes may also be present. Such problems can be mistaken for selfishness or awkwardness.

4. *Planning*
   Working out what steps are needed to put ideas into action can be difficult. People can seem to never get round to putting their ideas into practice or doing things they say they will do. Breaking tasks down into small steps can be very difficult. Problems in thinking through actions before doing them may also be present and show up as impulsivity. This can be mistaken for carelessness.

5. *Checking*
   Problems in 'standing back' and checking things out can occur. People can appear slapdash.

6. *Responding to social signals*
   People can have problems in learning through the advice and feedback of people around them. When with others, the less obvious signals that are used in conversations like suggestions, body language and smiles can be particularly difficult for people to notice

or use. As a consequence social rules may be broken more often, e.g. over-familiarity with strangers may occur because the rule about getting to know people slowly is not used or someone might be very talkative because the rule about taking turns in conversation is not followed. The person may also have reduced insight and awareness of their problems. They may therefore struggle to recognize when difficulties arise or accept help with them.

Particular Patterns of Problems

People with executive difficulties sometimes have particular patterns of problems. Some can tend to have most problems in acting without thinking, following social rules and inter-preting words and sentences in too many different ways. Others can tend to have problems getting themselves going, taking rules and regulations too seriously, and interpreting words and sentences in very literal ways, e.g. having dif-ficulties in understanding figures of speech and proverbs. These patterns of problems are like the opposite sides of the same coin when it comes to executive functioning.

Practical Things that May Help with Executive Problems

1. Breaking tasks down into small, logical steps. This can help provide the structure and planning with which the person may have problems. An example might be 'to make the sandwich you must i) get the bread, ii) find a knife, butter and jam, iii) butter the

bread, iv) spread jam on one of the slices and v) put the bread together'.

2. Using a diary to write down a structure and routine for each day and week. The diary should be carried and used at all times so that it becomes a habit to use it. This can help plan *what* to do each day, *when* to do it and *how* to do it. A diary is particularly important when someone has memory problems as well as executive ones.

3. Getting those who know the person well to ask multiple-choice questions rather than open-ended ones. An example might be 'Would you rather go to the shops or swimming tomorrow?' rather than 'What would you like to do tomorrow?' This can make it easier to make a decision.

4. Getting those who know the person well to tell them or signal to them when they are breaking social rules, e.g. when they need to stop talking because someone else is ready to say something. This can give valuable feedback about social rules. It *must only* be done when the person and others agree to it and when one specific social rule for feedback has been agreed upon.

5. Using a watch with an alarm, mobile phone 'alarm/reminder' function or a paging device as a cue to look at a diary and initiate particular tasks.

6. Using notes, calendars and lists as external cues to help initiate tasks.

7. Undertaking problem-solving skills training to help develop an explicit and systematic approach to

solving difficulties, e.g. i) defining the problem to be overcome; ii) generating different strategies to overcome the problem; iii) highlighting the pros and cons of each strategy; iv) deciding the best strategy based on the pros and cons; v) implementing the strategy; and vi) evaluating the outcome.

8. Using an alarmed stopwatch/mobile phone to help monitor the amount of time taken on given tasks to help planning and time-judgement impairments.

9. Talking to oneself about a task (verbal mediation) to help overcome initiation problems and to be reminded of any self statements that help social awareness.

10. Introducing repeated routines/cycles to reduce unnecessary decision-making (e.g. weekly menus, shopping lists, set times for visiting the gym, etc.).

Cognitive Rehabilitation Principles

In addition to the specific strategies that can help the common thinking problems, general cognitive rehabilitation principles can also be very important in achieving the best possible coping skills. Because the brain is not like a muscle, exercising a particular part of the brain using mental exercises usually makes very little difference to a person's real-life functioning. They are likely to improve their performance on the specific exercise being undertaken but are unlikely to gain any improved cognitive ability. Having said this, it is important to maintain a reasonable level of mental stimulation to keep mental health optimal but without 'overdoing it', which can lead to fatigue, irritability, stress or depression. The main focus in cognitive rehabilitation therefore is in developing a detailed understanding of the person's individual strengths and weaknesses in their thinking skills and creatively finding alternative practical ways of achieving the best day-to-day functioning.

Cognitive Rehabilitation Strategies

There are three important principles that substantially help to achieve optimal cognitive rehabilitation.

1. *Reducing 'mental load'*

    A large number of factors can cause the brain to work on 'reduced capacity'. These include post-concussion symptoms, stress, pain, anxiety, fatigue and brain injury. This is like a car running on three cylinders instead of four. In other words, the brain is constantly working harder than it would normally do. Everyday tasks therefore use up much more mental energy than before. This means that it is much easier to become mentally 'overloaded'. The most effective way of managing this problem is by reducing the 'mental load' on the brain. This can be done by:

    a) taking lots of small breaks during the day;
    b) using routines and familiar or 'autopilot' tasks as much as possible;
    c) undertaking small, achievable goals one at a time rather than altogether;

d) maintaining a good balance between resting and mental stimulation;

e) developing daily and weekly routines that involve meaningful daytime activities, e.g. voluntary work;

f) using practical 'compensatory' strategies to get around cognitive difficulties, e.g. using a diary for day-to-day memory difficulties;

g) returning to activities slowly and in small steps (progressing to each new step only when the previous step has been achieved);

h) minimizing self-criticism and self-blame regarding any difficulties caused by the mild traumatic brain injury;

i) avoiding taking on too many activities and responsibilities at any one time (this may involve learning to say 'No' more effectively).

2. *Mood management*

Emotional reactions like frustration, anger, irritability, loss of confidence, stress, anxiety and depression are very normal when managing cognitive difficulties. These emotional reactions, however, can make cognitive difficulties worse. Whilst this is not physically harmful it can lead to a vicious cycle where cognitive difficulties are made worse by emotional reactions, which then lead to greater cognitive difficulties etc. Alongside this, it is important to know that the process of adjusting to such problems often involves difficult emotions and is a slow process. Some people view it as a kind of emotional journey involving challenges along the way but with positive emotional growth occurring as understanding, insight and realistic hope are developed. For some this involves accepting at least part of themselves as being a 'new person'. This means that while they are the same person as before, they learn to accept some different characteristics in their make-up.

3. *Acceptance*

Two key elements of cognitive rehabilitation are:

a) understanding and accepting limitations;
b) finding practical ways to get around these diffi-culties.

Finding practical solutions to problems is often called 'compensation' and is far more effective than trying to restore lost thinking skills through mental exer-cises. Often people can push themselves to exhaus-tion in order to try to 'get back to normal' as soon as possible. This, however, often feels like 'wearing a mask' or 'putting on a brave face' when the per-son is actually struggling inside. It can be a relief to acknowledge this and 'take off the mask' to begin adjusting to things more openly.

This can sometimes be slowed down by the natural process of 'denial', which can help protect a person from having to work through difficult issues until they are ready to do so. It often takes some time to fully understand, accept and adjust to limitations. Being able to talk openly with someone about these things can help enormously. It can also be very beneficial for the person to have realistic (but supportive) feedback about their strengths and weaknesses from those close to them.

Case Study

Andy, a twenty-one year-old geography student suffered a mild traumatic brain injury as the result of being knocked off his bicycle on the way to lectures one morning. After being discharged from Accident and Emergency he was aware that he felt extremely fatigued and 'spaced out'. He had three weeks recuperation back home with his parents before returning to university. Although his symptoms had improved, once he tried studying again he quickly noticed that he was remembering very little from lectures or his reading and he was forgetting important appointments with his tutors. He also found himself struggling to stay awake in tutorials and did not have enough energy to keep on top of his role as secretary of the university badminton team, which he had previously really enjoyed. What most concerned him, though, was his 'brain just switching off' in conversations: although he was vaguely aware that someone was talking, 'nothing was going in'. These difficulties started to cause him a lot of worries about whether he would ever get sufficiently better to re-engage with his studies as he was falling further and further behind with his course assignments.

He eventually sought help from his general practitioner who managed to get him seen quickly by the local Brain Injury Service. He was seen by a brain injury nurse specialist and an occupational therapist who helped him understand what he was experiencing and to put into place some cognitive rehabilitation strategies. These included: recording lectures and writing them up afterwards; using the diary function on his mobile phone to always remind him of appointments and key things he needed to remember on a day-to-day basis; taking lots of small breaks when studying even if he did not feel tired; eradicating all distractions when reading or writing (i.e. no background music and working in the library where he would not be distracted by friends or flatmates).

He quickly found that these strategies helped 'take the pressure off his mind' as he no longer worried so much about his poor memory as it was now 'backed up' with his phone and lecture recordings. He also found that writing things down actually helped his memory and that he relied on his phone less over time. He said it was like 'having two bites of the cherry' to get things to stick in his memory – the first 'bite' when he was told something he needed to remember and the second 'bite' when he wrote it down in his phone. He found himself getting back on top of his studies and worrying much less about his problems. Six months after the accident he had caught up with all his course work and felt

'100 per cent better'. He carried on using his phone-diary as a memory aid as he had found it so useful and he now just did it 'on autopilot'.

Emotional Difficulties

There are many ways of understanding emotional difficulties after a mild traumatic brain injury. These types of problems can be part of the post-concussion symptoms themselves (e.g. depression, anxiety or irritability) or the result of trying to cope with the difficulties faced after the injury (e.g. the stress of having reduced cognitive resources) or the consequence of the traumatic nature of the injury-event (e.g. post-traumatic stress). The injury or injury-event can sometimes re-trigger past emotional problems that were previously resolved or worsen difficulties that were already present before. Also, there may be stressful and difficult life events or issues that emerge after the injury but are completely independent from it. These too can exacerbate emotional problems.

Cognitive Behavioural Therapy

One of the most useful ways of thinking about such problems and finding solutions to them is using **cognitive behavioural therapy (CBT)**. This breaks down our experience of things into four factors – **thoughts (cognitions), behaviour (actions), feelings (emotions) and bodily reactions (physical or biological responses)**. It is obvious that *some* of these factors influence each other, e.g. how we feel about something affects how we think about it. The powerful insight in CBT, however, is that *all* of the factors can affect *all* of the others, and in *all* directions. Therefore there are many different vicious cycles that can emerge and become mutually exacerbating. This can be summarized like this:

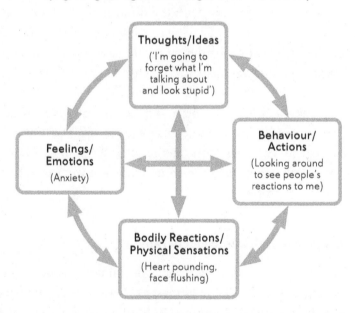

**CBT Diagram
(e.g. forgetting something in a conversation)**

Source: Adapted from C. A. Padesky, 1986 © www.mindovermood.com with permission of the copyright holder.

Cognitive behavioural therapy uses the simple but incredibly powerful idea that we can change our actions, thoughts or sometimes our bodily reactions to positively alter our feelings by transforming some of vicious cycles in the CBT Diagram into 'virtuous' ones.

The Most Common Emotional Difficulties

The most common emotional difficulties faced after a mild traumatic brain injury are anxiety/stress, depression, post-traumatic stress and irritability/anger. There is incredibly strong clinical evidence for how effective cognitive behavioural therapy can be in many of these kinds of problems and the following section outlines some of the ways they can be helped by CBT ideas. The 'Further Reading and Resources' section at the back of the book also lists just a few of the many CBT-based books that may be of further benefit in these areas. It is important to know that as well as the ideas in this book *there are many effective forms of medication which can be very helpful in these areas* and general practitioners, neurological physicians and psychiatrists are very knowledgeable about which might be of benefit for any individual.

The following sections are designed to be read on a 'pick and choose' basis depending on the specific areas that are relevant to the reader.

Anxiety and Stress

Anxiety and stress are often identical in nature and describe the feeling that arises in response to a real or perceived threat. Often this can be the threat that we are not going to be able to manage something because the perceived or actual demands we are facing are bigger than our perceived or actual resources. 'Threats' are often caused by difficult or worrying situations that we all face – they could be deadlines at work, arguments at home or trying to cope with new challenges, particularly if these are in response to major life changes such as adapting to persistent post-concussion symptoms. Feeling uptight, tense, jittery, apprehensive, on edge, panicky, fearful, worried or keyed up are different ways of describing the emotions of anxiety or stress.

Fight–Flight Response

When you are anxious or stressed, your body goes through a set of changes, which can be extremely helpful if you are facing a physical threat, as these changes enable your body and mind to be ready for action and respond quickly if necessary. This is a basic biological reaction to protect us from danger and is often called the 'fight-flight response' or 'increased arousal'. If you think about a caveman being faced with a wild animal, the body and mind have to prepare themselves to either fight the animal or run away (take flight). In today's terms this kind of response is vitally important when you step off the pavement and suddenly see a car about to hit you. Your fight-flight response helps you react quickly allowing you to jump out of the way. Without this response, you would not be able to respond quickly and get out of dangerous situations.

When Does Anxiety Become a Problem?

Many feelings of mild or short-acting anxiety are entirely healthy and we all need anxious responses at least from time to time to keep ourselves safe. In fact, moderate amounts of stress also improve our performance on many types of task, e.g. an applicant who did not feel some urgency before an interview could not expect to perform at his or her best.

The graph below is called the Yerkes Dodson curve and demonstrates this. It shows how well people perform tasks when experiencing low, medium or high anxiety. As you can see people perform many tasks best when stress levels are moderate, but at low or high levels, performance drops. Indeed, after a certain level of anxiety, people become unable to cope.

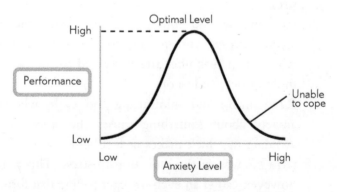

Source: Adapted from R. M. Yerkes and J. D. Dodson, 'The relation of strength of stimulus to rapidity of habit-formation', *Journal of Comparative Neurology and Psychology*, 18 (1908), 459–82.

Anxiety becomes a problem if it occurs when there is no real danger or when it goes on long after the threat is over. When anxiety begins to interfere with your everyday life, or affects your performance in important areas of day-to-day functioning, then it may be a problem for which you should seek help.

Remember, *anxiety is a normal, healthy reaction* that we cannot get rid of completely, but we can learn to manage it so it doesn't interfere with our lives.

What Helps?

The three key CBT principles to help with anxiety relate to the behaviour, thoughts and bodily reactions listed earlier:

1. Recognizing and reducing the cycle whereby *physical reactions* caused by an overactive fight-flight response lead to symptoms that cause us further worry and stress

2. Recognizing and minimizing the cycle whereby anxiety causes our *thinking* to become distorted, which then magnifies the perceived threat causing more anxiety and so on.

3. Recognizing and minimizing the cycle whereby anxiety about something causes the *action* of us avoiding it, which makes us feel better in the short term because of the reduction in stress. This relief, however, causes an even stronger feeling that further avoidance is the only way of managing the next time and so on. This is called behavioural reinforcement.

Physical Reactions

Because anxiety and stress are responses to a threat, our bodies prepare themselves to face up to the threat by getting ready to fight it or take flight from it: the fight-flight response. In order to do this, the body must direct all its energy to where it is needed. To make these changes, the body automatically releases a hormone called adrenaline. This speeds up bodily processes to direct more oxygen and energy to where it will be needed for us to fight or escape. Other chemicals are also released to slow down bodily processes that will be less useful in these types of situations.

When our bodies prepare to fight or take flight, the muscles, especially the major ones, such as in the back, neck and leg, tense up. This can cause them to feel shaky and sore. Keeping the muscles in this state requires extra glucose and oxygen, which occurs by the heart pumping much faster and the breathing quickening. All of these extra processes raise the body temperature so to cool it we sweat more and our cheeks may redden (blush), as the blood capillaries rise to the surface to get rid of excess heat. The body will also divert the glucose and oxygen supply from places it doesn't need for fighting. This is mainly the digestive system, so blood will be diverted away from the stomach, causing 'butterflies' and nausea. Less saliva is released in the mouth, making it dry, and as bladder muscles tense the urge to go to the toilet increases.

The physical symptoms that are common when you feel anxious are shown in the diagram below:

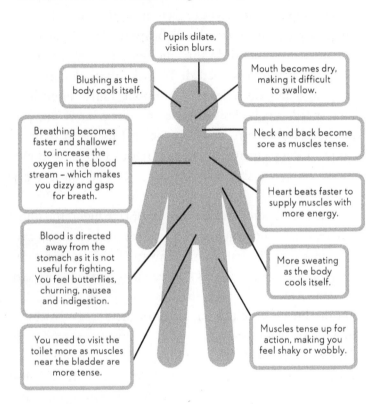

What Can I Do to Manage the Physical Reactions?

Controlled breathing techniques help reverse the physical fight-flight response and can be a very quick and effective way of tackling these elements of stress and anxiety. The flight-fight response causes the top of our chest area to do most of the work in our breathing. When stressed we automatically breathe more in this way, which causes more tension in our bodies. Relaxed breathing comes much more from the belly and abdomen area. If you sit or lie down and put your hands on your belly (a bit like pregnant women sometimes do when resting) you will be able to tell if you are breathing in a relaxed way or not. Your hands will be pushed slowly up and down as you breathe in and out if your breathing is relaxed.

How to Do Controlled Breathing:

A good way of quickly reducing anxiety levels is therefore to sit or lie down, place your hands on your tummy and take a deep, slow breath, making sure it comes from your belly and pushes your hands up as you do so. Breathe in slowly for a count of five, hold it for a count of three and then breathe out slowly for a count of five (making sure your hands on your tummy are being guided down as you do so). Concentrate on expelling most of the air in your lungs as you exhale. Repeat this for two to three minutes and you will quickly experience the calming effect of relaxed breathing. If you practise this for two to three minutes every day for three to four weeks you will soon be able to use it as a stress-management technique. It will also help to keep reminding you to regularly 'check in' with yourself over the course of the day to see if your breathing has become too tense.

Relaxation exercises also help reverse the physical fight-flight response. Some involve tensing and relaxing all the different muscle groups in your body slowly and system-atically. These are called *progressive muscle relaxation exercises* and can be very effective indeed. The resources at the end of the book show where you can get written instructions about this kind of exercise. They are, however, often best done with the help of a clinician and an audio recording to take away and use for practice. Other relaxation exercises rely more on our imagination but can also be very helpful. These too are best undertaken with a clinician and an audio recording. With regular practice these types of exercises can be very powerful stress-management techniques.

Physical exercise can also be of great benefit as it is a healthy means of using the energy generated by the fight-flight response. It also results in a natural tensing and relaxing of our muscles (once we have stopped!) and releases endorphin chemicals in the brain, which have natural calming and stress-reduction effects. Regular exercise therefore can be another powerful type of stress-management strategy.

Finally, just by understanding that the physical symptoms of anxiety are normal and not harmful and being able to control them better may help. This is because the vicious cycle (of stress symptoms causing worry about the symptoms causing more stress symptoms, etc.) is reduced.

Changes in Thinking

As well as preparing you for physical action, stress and anxiety prepare you to fight or escape mentally.

When people are anxious they tend to:

- worry about things before they actually happen;

- predict and expect the worst outcome of a situation;

- tell themselves that they will not be able to cope;

- become increasingly over-sensitized to the thing they are anxious about by unconsciously over-focusing their attention on it.

These lead to unhelpful thought patterns that usually operate outside of the person's awareness. These are termed *Negative Automatic Thoughts* (NATS) and the first step to helping is to become much more aware of them when they are occurring. Some typical examples of these include:

- *All or nothing thinking* – Viewing a situation in only two ways, i.e. in black-and-white categories and without any shades of grey: 'Because I'm afraid of driving I'll never be independent.'

- *Over-generalizing* – Making sweeping conclusions that go far beyond the current situation: 'If I don't know the answer to a question everyone will think I am stupid.'

- *Eliminating the positive* – Telling yourself that positive things don't count: 'I only managed to go to the shopping centre for the first time because my friend came with me.'

- *'Should statements'* – Having a precise idea of what should be done or how you should behave and telling yourself how bad it is if you don't live up to these expectations: 'I should be able to speak in public.'

- *Catastrophizing* – Predicting the worst outcome without considering more likely ones: 'If I don't face up to my fear of flying my partner will leave me.'

- *Emotional reasoning* – Thinking something is true because you feel it and discounting evidence to the contrary: 'I feel stupid so I must be stupid.'

- *Mind reading* – Thinking you *know* what others are thinking and not considering other possibilities: 'People think I'm unfriendly because I didn't talk to them.'

- *Personalization* – Thinking that other people's behaviour is solely due to you and not other factors: 'That person left the party because I said something they didn't like.'

- *Fortune telling* – Thinking you *know* how something will turn out in the future without trying it out: 'I know I'll get tongue-tied if I talk to someone I don't know very well.'

Source: Adapted from D. Burns, 'Thinking styles', in *Feeling Good: The New Mood Therapy* (New York: Morrow, 1980).

What Can I Do to Manage Changes in Thinking?

To help the person become more aware of these patterns, *thought records* are often used to record and notice when they are occurring, how intense they are and what triggers them. This is usually done for a few weeks before taking the next step of challenging them by considering alternative thoughts that are truer and more helpful.

Changes to Actions

When people experience anxiety, the natural reaction is to avoid getting into that anxious situation again. When people avoid situations they lose faith in their ability to do challenging things and this produces more anxiety. Avoiding something also reduces anxiety and discomfort in the short-term but only makes it harder to do the next time. This is because the positive feeling of relief acts like a 'reward' or 'reinforcement' for the avoidance behaviour, which then becomes self-reinforcing or self-rewarding.

What Can I Do to Manage Changes to Actions?

Generating a *behavioural hierarchy* is often the first step to helping this avoidance–reinforcement cycle. This involves making a very individualized 'ladder' of avoided situations that cause different degrees of anxiety. Those that cause mild anxiety, but enough to avoid them, would be towards the bottom. Those with moderate anxiety would be in the middle and situations causing very severe anxiety would be at the top. Often with professional help the person would then *expose* themselves to the situation right at the bottom of the ladder and stick with this until the anxiety level peaked and then dropped *while they were still exposing themselves to it*. This might take many minutes and mean sticking with fear that feels 'unbearable' until it drops. The process would then be repeated many times over a number of weeks until that situation no longer caused significant anxiety. The person would then be said to be *habituated* to this situation, and then the next situation on the ladder would be tackled and so on.

Individual Capacity for Stress

Another helpful way to think about anxiety is to recognize that we all have a limit to the stress that our bodies can manage effectively. The amount you can cope with depends upon:

1. the number and size of the *demands* in your life;
2. the type of person you are and your own *capacity* for stress.

This can be illustrated by the 'tap and glass' analogy opposite.

Do not forget that your capacity for stress is individual. What makes you feel stressed or anxious may not affect other people to the same degree or may not have affected you so much in the past. Part of effective stress management may therefore be to reassess the demands you have and try to reduce them to make them more manageable. This may involve finding ways of saying 'no' to things or seeing what tasks you might be able to delegate to others. Sometimes it is your perception of demands that can be altered. For example, if you have a lot of 'Should' Negative Automatic Thoughts in your life this will give the perception that you have many important demands but that may not actually be the case. Similarly if you have developed NATS about your abilities, you may actually have more personal resources

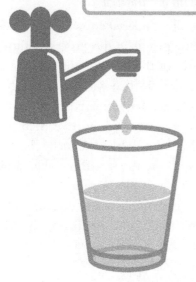

The Tap

These are stresses in our lives that turn the tap on, causing more stress. Something that may turn one person's tap on may not affect someone else's.

The Glass

We all have a different size stress-glass, i.e. an individual capacity for stress. So it may take less stress for someone with a small stress-glass to stop coping than someone with a large one. After a MTBI, some people find their stress-glass has become smaller, at least for a time, i.e. they cannot take as much stress in their lives.

The Water in the Glass

This represents the stress in your life. The more the glass fills, the more you will experience the symptoms of anxiety. Sometimes it can take only more more drip, one more small amount of stress, to cause someone's stress-glass to overflow. This is when you are no longer able to cope with stress in your life.

Source: Adapted from T. J. Powell and S. Enright, *Anxiety and Stress Management* (London: Routledge, 1990). Reprinted with permission.

than you have assumed. Tackling NATS may therefore be an additional way of helping your perceptions of demands and resources.

CBT on Your Own or with a Clinician

Usually CBT strategies are undertaken with a clinician with experience in helping people in this process: although the ideas behind this kind of therapy are not complicated they can be hard to put into practice without skilled help. Therefore do not think that CBT or other types of help will not be effective for you just because you have tried them on your own and they have not worked. Usually there is a huge difference between trying them without skilled help and trying them with it. It is a bit like learning to ride a bike for the first time – the ideas about how you do it are simple but they are very difficult to put into practice without the help of someone else.

Case Study

Caroline, a fifty-two-year-old primary school teacher, suffered a MTBI as the result of a road-traffic accident returning home from work one evening. She had a number of post-concussion symptoms including taking longer to think, reduced concentration, poor multi-tasking abilities and irritability. She felt under a great deal of pressure to return to work quickly as the school was finding it difficult to find a temporary teacher to take her class. She went back to full-time work after four weeks but had to put in huge amounts of effort to teach the children in her busy and sometimes noisy classroom. She was forgetting some of her pupils' names, making 'silly mistakes' (which were sometimes picked up by the children), avoiding meetings with parents and was putting in many extra hours work to try to cope with her responsibilities. She was exhausted by the end of the working week and spent a lot of weekends sleeping and resting with virtually no energy for social or family events.

Over a three-month period she found herself getting more and more anxious about her classroom abilities, noticing more and more 'silly mistakes' and having more and more days off work on sick leave. She stumbled across a friend's cognitive behavioural therapy self-help book, which she found very informative and helpful as she realized that a large number of Negative Automatic Thoughts had built up since her accident. She tried some of the thought-challenging strategies for her anxiety but did not have much success with them.

After seeing her general practitioner about her concerns she was referred to a CBT therapist. The therapist developed with Caroline a detailed and individualized explanation of her anxieties, how they had occurred over time and how some of them related to thinking patterns that had been around since her teenage years. They also discussed how some of her coping behaviours might have become 'part of the problem rather than part of the solution' to her stress and fatigue. Using thought monitoring and challenging with the therapist alongside exposure techniques, Caroline made great strides in overcoming her problems.

After eight weekly sessions she felt that her anxiety levels were 'under control'. She also became aware that a lot of the symptoms that were initially due to her MTBI had later been caused by her anxieties and that most of them had resolved as her anxiety had improved. She started to enjoy teaching again and she noticed that her increased energy levels meant that her social and family returned to 'life as usual'.

Additional very helpful information on cognitive behavioural therapy strategies for managing anxiety and stress can be found in two books in the same *Overcoming* series as this one, *Overcoming Anxiety* by Helen Kennerley and *Overcoming Stress* by Lee Brosan and Gillian Todd, and also *The Complete CBT Guide for Anxiety* edited by Roz Shafran, Lee Brosan and Peter Cooper.

Depression and Low Mood

Depression or low mood often describes the feeling we have in response to real or perceived losses. When people experience severe or prolonged problems after a mild traumatic brain injury they can often feel like they have lost their former self as they are not the person they used to be.

This might include the loss of important roles like being a breadwinner, a homemaker, a strong person, a helper of others, an extrovert or a good problem solver. There might also be more concrete losses like the ability to go out, make money or enjoy social relationships as much as before.

Physical symptoms like waking up early in the morning and being unable to get back to sleep, poor appetite, reduced interest in sex, low energy levels, fatigue, comfort eating and being restless or fidgety can all be symptoms of depression. *Thoughts* about how hopeless things are, having a very pessimistic view of the world, thinking about death and suicide, having ideas about low self-worth, engaging in self-critical and guilty thinking or believing that nothing will bring any pleasure are all common forms of depression-related cognitions (i.e. mental actions). *Feeling* sad, 'blue', numb, irritable, angry, empty, tense or bleak are often the emotions that people describe. Doing much less, e.g. just lying in bed or sitting in a chair a great deal, withdrawing from social activities and performing tasks much more slowly are the kinds of changes in *behaviour* that frequently occur.

If these types of difficulties are around nearly every day for a consistent period without going away, e.g. for at least two weeks, and they cause significant difficulties in the person's day-to-day functioning then 'clinical depression' or a 'major depressive disorder' might be the terms to describe these problems.

What Helps?

The three key CBT principles to help with depression relate to the behaviour, thoughts and bodily reaction factors listed earlier:

1. Recognizing and minimizing the *physical* changes caused by depression. We need a moderate amount of activity in our lives to keep our energy at normal levels. When we are depressed our energy levels feel lower and we end up doing less and less. In the end we are doing so little that our lack of activity prevents us from returning to normal energy levels. Strange as it sounds, this means we can get to a point where the less we do the more tired we get. We also become under-stimulated by doing less, particularly if we are staying indoors all the time. These can cause many vicious cycles to develop related to tiredness, demotivation and fatigue.

2. Recognizing and minimizing the *behavioural changes* caused by doing much less. The less we do the fewer experiences we have of pleasure or achievement. This means we have fewer and fewer rewarding experiences and less and less motivation to try any other positive and enjoyable things.

3. Recognizing and minimizing the cycle whereby depression causes our *thinking* to become distorted, which then magnifies the perceived losses, hopelessness and pessimistic ideas, causing more depression and so on.

Physical and Behavioural Changes

Doing less and less eventually makes us more and more fatigued and less fit. It also provides us with fewer and fewer self-rewarding experiences. For example, forcing ourselves to go to the café for a coffee and finding some enjoyment in doing so makes it more likely that we will go again the next time. Conversely not going and therefore not experiencing a positive feeling makes it more likely that we will not go the next time. Slowly increasing gentle *physical exercise* can therefore help fatigue levels and tiredness.

Activity scheduling can also help us understand the small things we already do that give us a small sense of pleasure or achievement. It can then help us to schedule more of these kinds of things into our weekly routines.

The first step is to keep a record of all the things that you do in each hour over a week or two. Although it can feel like 'I do nothing at all' this is actually impossible. 'Sleeping', 'sitting in a chair', 'making a cup of tea' and 'watching television' are all examples of the types of things we are actually doing when it feels like we are doing nothing at all. After each recording the person rates from 0 to 10 how *pleasurable* the activity was (their 'P' score) and how much *achievement* they gained from it (their 'A' score). This then gives some clear guidance as to how to slowly build up positive activities over time and reverse the vicious cycles caused by behavioural deactivation. Hourly records are usually continued until a solid routine of positive activity is completely bedded into weekly schedules.

Changes to Thinking

Unhelpful thought patterns, usually operating outside of the person's awareness will occur when they experience low mood. Like unhelpful anxious thoughts these are termed *Negative Automatic Thoughts* (NATS). The first step to helping them is to become much more aware of them when they are occurring. Some typical examples of these include:

- *All or nothing thinking* – Viewing a situation in only two ways, i.e. in black-and-white categories and without any shades of grey: 'Because I can't go to the shops on my own I am useless.'

- *Over-generalizing* – Making sweeping conclusions that go far beyond the current situation: 'Because I didn't go out on my own today I'll never be able to.'

- *Eliminating the positive* – Telling yourself that positive things don't count: 'I went for a walk on my own but only for ten minutes.'

- *'Should statements'* – Having a precise idea of what should be done or how you should behave and telling yourself how bad it is that you don't live up to these expectations: 'I should clean the house every day.'

- *Catastrophizing* – Predicting the worst outcome without considering more likely ones: 'If I don't finish my work today, I'll get sacked.'

- *Emotional reasoning* – Thinking something is true because you feel it and discounting evidence to the contrary: 'I feel embarrassed so I must be an idiot.'

- *Mind reading* – Thinking you *know* what others are thinking and not considering other possibilities: 'People think I'm unsociable because I didn't go out with them.'

- *Personalization* – Thinking that other people's negative behaviour is solely due to you and not other factors: 'My husband snapped at me because I am a failure.'

- *Fortune telling* – Thinking you *know* how something will turn out in the future without trying it out: 'I know I won't be able to successfully fix my bike so I won't.'

Source: Adapted from D. Burns, 'Thinking styles', in *Feeling Good: The New Mood Therapy* (New York: Morrow, 1980).

The unhelpful thought patterns when someone is low in mood tend to relate to ideas about low self-worth, hopelessness and punishment. Common examples include 'I'm a failure', 'This is a punishment that I deserve', 'There is no point to anything', 'I'll always be like this' and 'Nothing can be done to make me feel any happier'. To help the person become more aware of these patterns *thought records* are often used to record and notice when they are occurring, how intense they are and what triggers them. This is usually done for a few weeks before taking the next step of challenging them by considering alternative thoughts that are truer and more helpful.

Cognitive Behavioural Therapy on Your Own or with a Clinician

Usually CBT strategies are undertaken with a clinician with experience in helping people in this process: although the ideas behind this kind of therapy are not complicated they can be hard to put into practice without skilled help. Therefore, do not think that CBT or other types of help will not be effective for you just because you have tried them on your own and they have not worked. Usually there is a huge difference between trying them without skilled help and trying them with it. It is a bit like learning to ride a bike for the first time – the ideas about how you do it are simple but they are very difficult to put into practice without the help of someone else.

Additional very helpful information on CBT strategies for managing depression can be found in another book in the same *Overcoming* series as this one: *Overcoming Depression* by Paul Gilbert.

Post-traumatic Stress

After a disturbing or traumatic event, particularly one that is life threatening, people can experience a very distress-ing and frightening reaction. Sometimes this reaction is so intense it can be called post-traumatic stress. Unfortunately many of the situations where people sustain a MTBI are also those that are emotionally very traumatic, e.g. road-traffic accidents, violent encounters or any circumstances where the person thought they were about to die or be permanently disabled.

Post-traumatic Stress (PTS)

PTS is a deep emotional response to an intensely traumatic experience. It results in the person re-experiencing many of the painful feelings and memories that occurred at the time of the trauma. These can take the form of nightmares, flashbacks, intrusive memories or images, feeling like the person is reliving the event or distressing feelings when things bring the event to mind. Sometimes these are particularly powerful or more frequent when first waking up or when intoxicated.

Avoidance

Often the painful feelings cause people actively to avoid things that remind them of the event and to avoid thinking or talking about it altogether.

Anxiety

Deep feelings of anxiety and fear are common in PTS and often people feel very alert or 'on their toes' for long periods of the day. It often feels like the threat at the time of the event is still very much current and in the 'here and now' rather than in the past. Sleeplessness, poor concentration, forgetfulness and irritability are also common.

Thoughts

Traumatic and life-threatening events can powerfully contradict and call into question very basic and important assumptions about life and how predictable, controllable and safe it is. Post-traumatic stress can therefore make the person see the world as a much more dangerous and hazardous place. The future can feel much less optimistic and seem like it is not worth planning for because it is so unpredictable. Fewer things can seem like they are under the person's control or make sense to them. Consequently people can become much more inward-looking, less interested in the things that were once important to them and much more negative about how they view themselves.

Feelings

Alongside intense fear and anxiety people with PTS commonly have feelings of emptiness and numbness. Others have feelings of guilt about having survived the event or even about how they behaved during it. Sometimes people feel very angry about the cause of the trauma, particularly if it was someone else's fault. Feelings of depression, irritability or shame are also often present.

Some General Advice

1. *Don't* bottle up feelings. Do try to express your emotions to your close family and friends.
2. *Don't* expect the memories to go away suddenly. It takes time for the feelings to become less intense.

3. *Don't* rely on alcohol, drugs or smoking to cope.
4. *Do* talk about what happened. Take every opportunity to review the experience within yourself and with others.
5. *Do* give yourself time to sleep, rest, think and be with your close family and friends.
6. *Do* express your needs clearly and honestly to family, friends and officials.
7. *Do* drive more carefully and be more careful around the home: accidents are more common after severe stresses.

Post-traumatic Stress Disorder

When PTS symptoms are particularly strong and have not got better over time they may be termed post-traumatic stress disorder (PTSD).

When to Seek Professional Help

1. If you feel you are struggling to manage your intense feelings or bodily sensations.
2. If you feel that your emotions are not falling into place over a period of time, you are avoiding many things to stop feelings of fear/anxiety or if you feel persistent confusion, emptiness or exhaustion.
3. If you continue to feel numb and empty or have to keep active in order not to feel.
4. If you continue to have nightmares, flashbacks or poor sleep.

5. If your relationships or your job are suffering.
6. If you have accidents or continue to smoke, drink or take drugs to excess in order to cope.
7. If you think that your problems constitute PTSD.

What Help Would You Get?

Because of the intensely distressing nature of the feelings involved in PTS, it is often very difficult for people to seek help. Medication and/or specialist counselling, however, can both be extremely effective in treating PTS. Medication can help reduce the intensity of the symptoms and aid sleep. Specialist counselling may be of benefit in the following ways:

1. by explaining in detail how your specific trauma relates to your specific problems;
2. by looking, with you, at the thoughts, feelings and behaviours that you have that help or hinder the healing process;
3. by helping to process the very strong feelings and reduce their intensity;
4. by advising on practical ways that can further help your specific feelings and problems, and to slowly reclaim back normality.

Case Study

Colin, a sixty-six year-old retired mechanic, suffered a mild traumatic brain injury as the result of a high-speed,

*side-impact, road-traffic accident. He escaped with rela-
tively minor injuries – a badly bruised chest and a whiplash neck injury. There was, however, a brief moment just
before the other car hit his vehicle when he was convinced
he was going to be killed. He was seen in Accident and
Emergency and discharged the same day having been told
that he had sustained a minor head injury and a whiplash
injury. After two or three days of sleeping a great deal,
experiencing high levels of pain and 'just feeling dead to
the world', he started to notice quite severe problems with
anxiety, nightmares about the accident (where it felt like
he was exactly reliving the moment when he thought he
was about to be killed), 'excruciating' headaches, neck
pain, 'terrible concentration' and irritability.*

*There was a short period where he thought some of
these problems were getting a bit better but as he tried
to 'return to normal' he found them getting worse and
worse. He stayed in more and more due to his anxieties; his relationship with his wife became strained due
to his short fuse (and both of them not understanding
why he was behaving as he was); he avoided watching
any television programmes that might involve car crashes
or hospitals; he became more and more withdrawn in
himself; he slept badly because of the nightmares and
neck pain; he was scared to go to sleep each night in case
he experienced a nightmare; he was unable to be a car
passenger and could only drive short distances on very
familiar routes due to driving anxieties; he was less and
less able to concentrate on his hobbies; and he found it*

harder and harder to help out looking after his grandchildren with his partner. He felt 'like he was going mad'.

He spoke to his general practitioner who referred him to the local Brain Injury Service. He was eventually seen two-and-a-half months later by a clinical neuropsychologist. After a thorough assessment they discussed together how his problems may at first have involved some post-concussion symptoms from the MTBI but probably now resulted from a combination of post-traumatic stress disorder (PTSD) and whiplash neck pain. These had led to a number of vicious cycles, which meant that his symptoms had got worse rather than better over time. This explanation 'fitted' for Colin and immediately helped him understand what was causing his difficulties and that he was not 'going mad'. This in itself helped ease some of his difficulties a little.

Over the next nine months, he had specialist counselling with the clinical neuropsychologist to help him process the powerful feelings of fear and anxiety he was experiencing and to slowly reduce his avoidance of things and conversations that reminded him of the accident. Antidepressant medication from his GP also helped his anxiety, sleep and pain. He saw a physiotherapist who gave him some exercises to help his whiplash pain and he also used some pain-management techniques to help distract himself when it was at its worse. By one year after the accident he felt that he was '95 per cent recovered' and he wanted to carry on managing his residual symptoms without professional help. He was therefore

> *discharged from the Brain Injury Service but on the basis that he could re-refer himself back in the future if any 'booster sessions' were needed.*

Additional very helpful information on cognitive behavioural therapy strategies for managing post-traumatic stress can be found in another book in the same *Overcoming* series as this one: *Overcoming Traumatic Stress* by Claudia Herbert and Ann Wetmore.

Irritability and Anger

It is normal to feel angry or irritable sometimes. Anger can be a positive emotion, e.g. it can motivate us to correct a wrong.

It becomes a problem when it:

- occurs too frequently;
- is too intense or out of proportion to the situation;
- lasts too long;
- leads to aggression.

Irritability can often occur when your cognitive and emotional demands have started to outweigh your internal resources. As these can be significantly reduced if you are experiencing PCS it is usually an essential starting point to carefully evaluate whether demands have increased over time. This can often happen very slowly and imperceptibly over a long period of time. A useful thing to do is to think back to a time when the irritability was less of a problem and gauge whether you have now taken on more responsibilities, tasks or activities (even if they are enjoyable ones). If you have then the information on pages 30–33, which highlights the differences in demands and resources, may help readjust things and quickly improve irritability or anger problems.

If irritability is still a problem after you have done this, the following strategies might also be helpful:

Understanding Anger and How it Occurs

Anger and irritability often feel like they happen 'out of the blue' and we can feel like we 'just snap'. *However, usually there are warnings and triggers that we can learn to spot.*

Anger and irritability involve your mind and your body and you may over time have developed unhelpful ways of reacting to situations that make you angry.

Ways to Manage Irritability

1. *Learn to recognize the triggers*
   - There is usually a pattern to your anger. It may tend to happen in particular situations, with particular people and with particular provocations, e.g. hunger, tiredness, noise, alcohol, traffic, crowds, being ignored, etc.
   - Keep a diary recording a) where you were; b) who was there; c) what was going on each time you get angry.

Trigger

There is usually an event or situation
(sometimes relatively minor)
which acts as a trigger.

We interpret the event/situation

Thoughts go through our heads and we
put our own 'slant' on the situation.

This leads to a particular point of view:

- We feel we are being treated unfairly

- We feel we are being hurt unnecessarily

- We feel rules have been broken

- We are prevented from achieving a goal
  we have set

We have a physiological reaction:

Our skin temperature, heart and pulse rate rise.
The hormone, adrenaline, is released, preparing our bodies for 'fight or flight'.

This leads to physical responses:

- Muscles becoming tense
- Feeling hot/cold
- Going red in the face
- Chills and shudders
- Goosebumps
- Feeling nauseous
  or sick
- Breathing becoming
  shallow and fast

- Scowling
- Glaring
- Grinding teeth
- Clenching fists
- Sweating
- Choking

- You will notice it is usually not random and not an 'uncontrollable force'.

2. *Identify what is upsetting you*
   - What is it about the situation that you find annoying/irritating?
   - What are you thinking when these situations occur?
   - Make a list of the kinds of statements that go through your mind. Try to come up with alternative ways of looking at the situation that make you less angry.

3. *Recognize the physical signs or 'warning signs'*
   - Pay attention to your body and notice if you have any of the signs mentioned in the diagram on page 117, e.g. clenched fists, gritted teeth.
   - Practise deep-breathing exercises which will combat the physical reaction (see 'What Can I Do to Manage the Physical Reactions?' on pages 92–94).

4. *Anticipate and prepare*
   - Once you become aware of the kinds of situations where you are more likely to become irritable and angry you can prepare for them.
   - Practise what you are going to say and how.
   - Watch for the physical signs and breathe deeply.
   - Be aware of the thoughts running through your mind and replace unhelpful thoughts with more helpful ones.

5. *Time out*
   - If you feel your anger is getting out of control *remove yourself from the situation.*
   - 'Cool off' – count to ten, sleep on it, distract yourself, exercise or relax.

6. *Manage overall stress levels*
   - High levels of stress over time can cause anger and frustration.
   - Lowering stress levels will give you a greater 'buffer zone'.
   - Exercise regularly.
   - Set aside time for relaxation.
   - Look at your lifestyle.

7. *Discuss and explore feelings*
   - Do not 'bottle up' feelings until you 'explode'.
   - Talk to friends and family, or discuss issues with a professional if necessary.

8. *Avoid 'bad habits'*
   - Avoid yelling, sulking, plotting revenge, violence, accusations and arguing while angry.

9. *Use cognitive behavioural therapy (CBT) techniques*
   - Challenge unhelpful thoughts like 'I should not be treated like that', 'How dare they behave like that', 'They are deliberately being difficult' (see 'Cognitive Behavioural Therapy' on page 85 onwards).

Case Study

Christopher, a twenty-nine-year-old office cleaner, suffered a MTBI one night as the result of a heavy piece of cleaning equipment falling on his head from a high shelf at work. He was initially quite confused and extremely frightened: while he was 'coming round' he experienced very severe dizziness and head pains and he thought he was going to die with no one else in the building to help him. From day one he experienced a large number of severe post-concussion symptoms. These included poor concentration and short-term memory problems as well as nightmares about the accident. He also avoided talking about the accident.

After two months he had been unable to return to night duties, was only working a few hours a week and found himself increasingly irritable and angry. His wife and six-year-old son often bore the brunt of his outbursts and he felt extremely guilty after each one, but he felt as though they came completely 'out of the blue' and were 'pretty much uncontrollable'. Twelve months after the accident he had managed to return to work half-time but was still not doing any night duties. He was still very irritable and 'snappy' and this was causing a lot of strain in his relationship with his wife. He felt he had 'completely changed as a person' and hated the 'new' man he had become.

After seeing his general practitioner he was referred to a clinical neuropsychologist, and they discussed together how both PCS and post-traumatic stress were combining to cause his difficulties, which were made worse by the worry and anxiety about his anger difficulties and his sense of being 'out of control'. Treatment first focused on some specialist post-traumatic stress counselling to help him process his powerful feelings of fear and anxiety and to slowly reduce his avoidance of things and conversations that reminded him of the accident. Relaxation exercises were then introduced. Christopher practised these every day and they helped not only reduce his overall tension levels but made him much more sensitive to when tension or irritability were slowly building up, rather than just 'exploding out of the blue'. This meant that he could increasingly anticipate when he needed to withdraw from a situation that was causing him anger or to count to ten in his head so that he had 'more room in his mind' to think of calmer ways of viewing the situation. This made him feel like he had a 'much longer fuse' and was more in control of himself.

He also realized that his life demands were too much for the reduced resources he had. He therefore discussed things with his wife and reduced some of his domestic responsibilities. He learnt to say 'no' a bit more when friends asked him to take on things he felt unable to complete. This gave him a greater sense of control in his weekly routines. He was eventually able to resume night duties and full-time work, and his relationship with his son and wife improved significantly (particularly after his wife joined a session to *gain a better understanding of his problems). Two years after the accident, Christopher's wife felt that he was 100 per cent better even though he was aware that he still used strategies to help him manage some of his residual feelings of irritability.*

Additional very helpful information on cognitive behavioural therapy strategies for managing irritability and anger can be found in another book in the same *Overcoming* series as this one: *Overcoming Anger and Irritability* by William Davies.

Physical Difficulties

The following sections are designed to be read on a 'pick and choose' basis depending on the specific areas that are relevant to the reader.

Headaches

Headaches are very common whether you have had a mild traumatic brain injury or not. It is extremely rare, however, that a headache means there is something wrong with your brain. In fact, we do not have any pain sensors in our brains and surgeons only need to anaesthetize the scalp when they perform brain surgery. After a MTBI the headaches may be caused or worsened by some of the small nerve-endings in your scalp being slightly damaged at the site of the injury, causing pain signals to be generated much more frequently and severely. Injuries to the neck can also affect the nerves running to the scalp and cause more frequent or intense pain signals in the head area. When more pain signals are sent, the scalp muscles become tenser, causing the nerves to be more aggravated and so on.

There are three main types of headache and over-the counter analgesics can often be very effective for them:

- *Tension-type headaches* are the most frequent form. These often have a dull aching sensation and can be made worse by stressful situations or tension. Most headaches after whiplash neck injuries are tension-type headaches.

- *Post-traumatic migraines* are rare but do sometimes occur. A migraine attack is often more severe than a tension headache. It is usually a throbbing headache and people frequently feel sick. Sometimes people have blurred vision, see flashing lights or are sensitive to light.

- *Cluster headaches* are also quite rare. They come on rapidly and are typically relatively short-lasting. Usually there is intense pain over the eyes and fore-head and the eyes might water.

Many people worry that their headaches mean there is something serious happening in the brain. Because this worry makes their scalp muscles tenser this actually makes the headaches worse and a vicious circle develops:

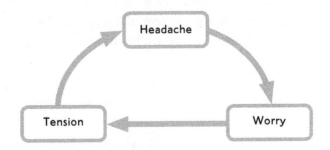

In most cases headaches do not mean anything serious at all. It is wise, however, to have frequent headaches checked out by your general practitioner as a precaution and they may be able to prescribe medication to help with the pain should over-the-counter treatments not work for you.

Coping with Headaches

Once you have found out about the cause of your headaches you do not have to worry unnecessarily each time you feel one coming on. The following strategies can also be very helpful in managing them:

- *Remind yourself* that the pain does not mean brain damage or physical harm.

- *Deep breathing and relaxation exercises* can help reduce the tension that may cause the headaches or make them worse (see 'What Can I Do to Manage the Physical Reactions?' on pages 92–94).

- *Exercise* releases endorphins, which are the body's natural painkillers. It also results in muscle relaxation.

- *Pacing* helps you avoid getting into a pattern where you do too much when you are feeling good and pay for it later! Spread out your activity with plenty of breaks. Try to have a mixture of physical and mental activity.

- *Distract yourself* by undertaking and paying attention to enjoyable activities or those that give you a sense of purpose and achievement (e.g. hobbies, DIY, voluntary work, DVDs, music). This can help you be less sensitive to your headache pain.

- *Use cognitive behavioural therapy techniques* (CBT) to challenge unhelpful thoughts like 'I can't cope', 'I'm a failure', 'I'll never be happy again' (see 'Cognitive Behavioural Therapy' on page 85 onwards).

Sleep

What Is a Good Night's Sleep?

A good night's sleep is not uninterrupted sleep. It is quite rare, in fact, to sleep without waking at some time in the night. As many as one in five people complain of difficulty in falling to sleep, waking too frequently during the night or waking too early in the morning. So it is not unusual to be concerned about your sleep pattern. Disturbed sleep, however, can sometimes become a problem, particularly when it becomes a worry. This, more than anything, can interfere with sleep and can leave you feeling exhausted the next day.

A Few Facts about Sleep that May Be Helpful

- Almost everyone has 'broken' sleep. The majority of people wake several times during the night and simply go back to sleep. When you worry about this happening you may notice and pay attention to the waking up more. This in turn can cause more worry and less sleep and so on.
- There is no such thing as an 'ideal night's sleep'. Some people need ten hours and others only three. If you sleep less than eight hours a night you are not necessarily depriving your body as you might not need eight hours.
- There is no danger in losing a few 'good night's sleep'. Everyone has the odd period of poor sleep, especially when under stress. The only ill effect of this is that you will feel tired during the day and might feel a bit more irritable or less able to cope with things.
- Sleep is affected by many things: stress, mood, exercise, illness, food, medicines, alcohol and worries. You may be able to solve your sleep problem by changing any of these.

Many people learn to sleep better without resorting to medication, simply by changing their behaviour. However, sleep patterns tend to change slowly. It may take a few weeks to establish a new pattern.

A Better Night's Sleep

There are two main approaches to preparing for a better night's sleep. Taken together they are often called having good *sleep hygiene*:

1. Tackling any physical problems to sleep

   - *Waking to use the toilet*: The need to urinate often disturbs our sleep. If this disturbs you then, first, make sure you empty your bladder just before you go to bed. Second, redistribute your drinking by limiting yourself to only a little during the evening, and drinking the rest before then. This does not mean drinking *less* but just changing the timing of when you do so.

   - *Cutting out stimulants*: People are affected differently by the stimulating effects of caffeine so you may have to experiment to find whether drinks and food with high levels of caffeine affect you and how close to bedtime you can have these. For many people avoiding all caffeine in tea, coffee, cocoa, chocolate, energy drinks and cola for approximately three to five hours before going to bed considerably helps their sleep. Try having a milky drink before bed instead. It should also be borne in mind that tobacco can act as a stimulant so avoiding smoking in the evening can help.

- *Alcohol*: Alcohol interferes with our sleep in two ways. First, it makes us want to go to the toilet more than usual. If you drink alcohol in the evening you may wake more during the night to pass urine or because you feel thirsty. Second, it has sedative effects. This means that it will send you to sleep at first but tends to wake you when the effects wear off. Moderating when and how much alcohol you drink may therefore help you sleep better.

- *Your bed*: Make sure that your bedroom is quiet, that your bed is comfortable and that the room temperature is to your liking. Ask yourself whether you get too hot or cold in bed over the course of a night, whether your bedding or bedclothes help you maintain a comfortable temperature and if opening the window or turning down the heating may help.

- *What you eat*: For some people sleeplessness is caused by changes in blood sugar levels at night. This can be tackled by avoiding eating sugary foods (e.g. puddings, sweets, biscuits) in the two to three hours before bed and replacing them with foods that release sugars slowly (e.g. cereals, porridge, pasta).

2. Establishing regular sleeping routines

We generally function best when we maintain good sleeping and waking routines. This is because we have natural biological cycles that our bodies prefer to work with rather than go against. *The most import-ant principle is to go to bed at the same time each night and to wake up at the same time each morning as much as is humanly possible.* Other important things to do include the following:

- *An evening routine*
  a) Make time to relax an hour or two before you go to bed. For example, go for a gentle walk, have a warm bath or sit and listen to sooth-ing music. Explain what you are doing to others so that they understand it. You may have to turn off your mobile phone, unplug your telephone or ask people not to call you once you have started your 'evening routine' of relaxing before you go to bed. Refrain from using your computer, gaming console, laptop or mobile phone for at least one to two hours before your allocated bedtime.
  b) It is recommended that your last meal should not be too large or too late. Avoid spicy food but do not go to bed hungry as this will keep you awake. Try having a light snack.
  c) Use your bedroom only for sleeping. Do not use it for eating, reading, using your mobile

phone, playing on your gaming console, being on your computer/laptop or watching TV. Some people, however, find quietly listening to music or the radio in the background when trying to get off to sleep helpful, particularly if it helps to distract them from worries or concerns going around their mind.

d) If you have not fallen asleep after 15–20 minutes, or if you have woken and not got back to sleep after 15–20 minutes, then get out of bed and do something light and not too stimulating until you feel sleepy – something simple like light housework, reading or watching the television. Then try to sleep again once you are feeling sleepy. Keep repeating this until you fall asleep rather than lying in bed tossing and turning.

- *A morning routine*
  a) Set an alarm and wake at a regular time each day. Get up when your alarm goes off and do not be tempted to catch up on your sleep during the day or through 'lie-ins' at the weekends.

  b) Avoid napping, as sleeping during the day may well interfere with your sleep at night.

  c) Keep your daily stress low. Make sure you are not overworking and that you are dealing with problems as they arise and not taking them to bed with you as worrying thoughts.

d) Take exercise during the day BUT not late in the evening as it is stimulating and arousing, and could keep you awake.

If you still have trouble sleeping once you have established good sleep hygiene for at least three to four weeks then it may be helpful to see your general practitioner to discuss whether any medication may help to 'kick-start' better sleep and sleep routines.

Case Study

Chloe, a forty-three year-old part-time sales assistant with two teenage daughters, suffered a mild traumatic brain injury as the result of a mountain bike accident. Even after three months she still felt 'muzzy-headed', slowed in her thinking, more irritable and very tired. Consequently she found it very difficult to get through her working days without feeling exhausted and stressed. As a result she often had a forty-five-minute nap in the afternoons. She had been a 'good sleeper' before the accident but ever since had found it really difficult to get off to sleep and to stay asleep throughout the night.

At first she carried on going to bed at her normal time of 11.30 p.m. but found that she did not get off to sleep for about two hours and then woke up two or three times during the night. She hardly ever woke up feeling refreshed. Over time she developed a habit of going to bed earlier, at 11 p.m., and texting and watching television in bed until she finally fell asleep, often not until 2.30 a.m. She still woke up a few times during the night but would lie-in until 10.30 a.m. on the days she was not working. Even sleeping longer in this way made no difference to how refreshed she felt and her daughters kept telling her she was getting increasingly 'ratty' and they were 'having to walk on eggshells' around her in the evenings.

She wondered whether her sleep problems were largely to blame for her symptoms and her general practitioner gave her a leaflet on 'Sleep Hygiene' to consider. She decided to change her sleep routines in the following ways:

1. *to go to bed at her normal time of 11.30 p.m. each night regardless of how tired she felt;*
2. *to set her alarm for her normal wake-up time of 7.30 a.m. and to get up at this time regardless of how she felt;*
3. *to stop all coffee, tea and chocolate after 5 p.m.;*
4. *to turn off her mobile and not use her computer after 9 p.m.;*
5. *to stop napping during the day;*
6. *if she had not got off to sleep after twenty minutes to get out of bed and quietly watch television in the lounge until she felt sleepy and then return to her bed.*

Within six weeks of using this routine her sleep had returned to very close to 'normal' and the majority of her symptoms had been completely resolved. She felt much more in control of her life and her daughters both commented that they had 'got their old mum back'.

Additional very helpful information on cognitive behavioural therapy strategies for managing sleep difficulties can be found in another book in the same *Overcoming* series as this one: *Overcoming Insomnia and Sleep Problems* by Colin Espie.

Pain

Difficult or chronic pain can occur for many reasons and approximately 10 per cent of people experience such difficulties at some point in their lives. Also, many pain-relief medications work best only when used occasionally and for immediate pain. They therefore become less and less effective when taken consistently for long-term pain. Before anything else it is important that a medical assessment has been undertaken to make sure that there are no undiagnosed medical reasons for the pain and that doing things that lead to pain will not cause any physical harm or injury.

Key Principles

Once all appropriate pain-relief medication and medical interventions have been considered the following *pain management strategies* should be attempted. The most important principle in these is to minimize three powerful vicious cycles:

1. pain causing muscle tension, causing more pain and so on;
2. pain causing reduced physical movements, causing muscle inflexibility, causing muscle tension, causing more pain and so on;
3. the thought that 'if I do something that causes me pain it will result in physical harm or injury', causing less activity, causing muscle inflexibility and low mood, causing more pain and so on.

Our experience of pain is also made worse by stress, depression, anger, sleeplessness and muscle tension, which causes more pain and so on. So anything that can reduce these factors may help to start 'virtuous cycles' rather than vicious ones. The following diagrams illustrate two of these cycles:

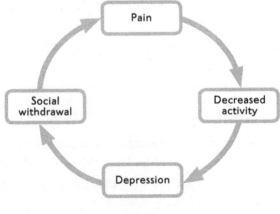

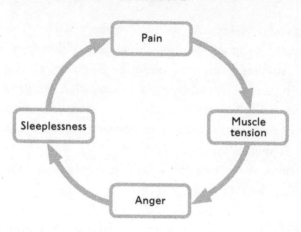

Another key principle is to avoid a 'boom-bust' approach to activities. This occurs when the pain feels a bit better and so we push ourselves to achieve more only to feel worse and experience a 'payback' the following day. This leads to us being able to do less the next day, feeling like we are behind with things, feeling like we are less in control of our life and our body and being more likely to overdo things again the next time our pain feels better. Pacing activities, taking regular breaks even if we are feeling pain free and keeping a moderate activity going consistently are more helpful than a 'boom-bust' approach. This will also allow you to increase the amount of time you spend on activities gradually and systematically (see below).

What Our Attention Is Focused On

Other difficulties occur when the pain becomes more and more the focus of our attention. This may cause you to become over-sensitive to it and make it worse. The more you can focus on positive things and undertake rewarding activities (even small ones) the better the pain will be. Setting and achieving realistic goals within the limitations of the pain, exercising regularly and using relaxation exercises can be vital elements in stopping vicious cycles from developing.

Some of the best ways to help manage pain therefore include the following:

- Gentle exercise such as walking, swimming and dancing can ease discomfort by blocking pain signals to the brain. Keeping mobile also helps reduce the contribution of muscle tension and inflexibility to pain.
- Use controlled breathing to breathe slowly and deeply when you feel pain start (see 'What Can I Do to Manage the Physical Reactions?' on pages 92–94). This helps our physical relaxation and keeps our muscles from tensing up and exacerbating the pain.
- Accept your limitations and pace your activities. This means having regular short rest periods on tasks even when you are pain-free to minimize difficulties due to a 'boom–bust' approach.
- Distract yourself by undertaking and paying attention to enjoyable activities or those that give a sense of purpose and achievement, e.g. hobbies, DIY, voluntary work, DVDs, music.
- Have a regular sleep routine to give you the best

chance of sleeping through the night. The section above on 'Sleep' might be helpful in this area.

- Set realistic goals to gradually increase the amount you do and restart the things that you have come to avoid. This should be done by first establishing a baseline amount of activity that you are able to do comfortably and that is completely sustainable over time. For example, you could establish how far you are able to walk before it is too painful and then reduce this distance by 20 per cent as your baseline level. You can then increase an activity by a small amount, e.g. 10 per cent, until this new level of activity feels comfortable and sustainable, just by sheer repetition. This may take a number of weeks or even months to achieve but you will then have a new baseline to work from. This process can then be repeated and continued.

- Keep in touch with friends and family and try to talk about anything other than your pain so that your attention is not overly drawn towards it.

- Relaxation techniques like anxiety management training or meditation can help to reduce the contribution of stress and muscle tension to the pain (see 'Anxiety and Stress' on page 88 onwards).

- About 10 per cent of people with chronic pain find that what they eat or drink is a factor. The most common nutritional causes of pain are alcohol, cheese, caffeine (in coffee, tea, cola, chocolate, cocoa or energy drinks), nuts or yoghurt. However, if you have an allergy to other foods like citrus fruits, wheat products or dairy products these might also contribute to your pain.

- Assess whether your posture when sitting, standing or walking is contributing to your pain. Your general practitioner or a physiotherapist will be able to advise you on the best postures to minimize pain if you are unsure about whether this is a factor for you.

- Use cognitive behavioural therapy techniques (CBT) to challenge unhelpful thoughts like 'I can't cope', 'I'm a failure' and 'I'll never be happy again' (see 'Cognitive Behavioural Therapy' on page 85 onwards).

Additional very helpful information on cognitive behavioural therapy strategies for managing pain can be found in another book in the same *Overcoming* series as this one: *Overcoming Chronic Pain* by Francis Cole, Helen Macdonald, Catherine Carus and Hazel Howden-Leach.

Fatigue

Difficult or chronic fatigue, like pain, can occur for many reasons. These include post-concussion symptoms, low mood, stress and chronic fatigue syndrome as well as a wide range of other medical conditions. A medical assessment should therefore be undertaken first to make sure that there are no undiagnosed medical reasons for it. Once all appropriate medication and medical interventions have been considered, the following *fatigue management strategies* should be attempted.

Key Principles

A key principle is to avoid a 'boom-bust' approach to activities. This occurs when the fatigue feels a bit better so we push ourselves to achieve more only to feel worse and experience a 'payback' the following day. This leads to us being less able to do as much, feeling behind with things, feeling less in control of our life and our body, and makes us more likely to overdo things again the next time our fatigue feels better. Pacing activities, taking regular breaks even if we are feeling energetic and keeping a consistent, moderate level of activity going are much more helpful than a 'boom-bust' approach. This will also allow you to increase the amount of time you spend on activities gradually and systematically from a stable foundation (see below).

Another important principle is to minimize the vicious cycle of fatigue causing you to struggle to manage day-to-day living causing stress and anxiety, leading to less refreshing sleep, leading to more fatigue and so on.

What Our Attention Is Focused On

A further principle is being aware that over time our thoughts and behaviours in relation to our fatigue can slowly change and add to the stress levels. This can involve us imperceptibly focusing our attention more and more on tiredness, avoiding more and more activities we previously found rewarding, and finding that the meaning the fatigue has in our lives has become more and more negative. All of these can add fuel to the vicious cycle of fatigue leading to stress, leading to more fatigue, etc.

Some of the best ways to help manage your fatigue therefore include the following:

- Accept your limitations and pace activities so that you have regular short rest periods on tasks even when you have more energy. This helps minimize difficulties caused by a 'boom-bust' approach.
- Set realistic goals to gradually increase the amount you do. This should be done by first establishing a basic amount of activity that you are able to do comfortably and that is completely sustainable over time. You can then increase an activity by a small amount, e.g. spending 10 per cent more time doing it, until this new level of activity feels comfortable and sustainable, just by sheer repetition. This may take a number of weeks or even months to achieve but then the process can be repeated and continued.
- Take regular gentle exercise such as walking, swimming and dancing. This can help increase energy levels and reduce stress.
- Establish a regular sleep routine. This will give you the best chance of sleeping through the night and minimize the effects of poor sleep on tiredness. The section on 'Sleep' in this book might be helpful in this area (see pages 125–33).
- Do routine and familiar tasks when fatigue and

concentration are 'at their worst' (e.g. at the end of an afternoon or end of a week).

- Do new and unfamiliar tasks when you are 'at your best' (e.g. in the morning or at the beginning of a week).
- Always use a diary to plan the day and pace yourself.
- Cut down on non-essential activity if it falls outside your current baseline level of activity. This may involve learning to say 'No' to things more – do not feel guilty about this.
- Use cognitive behavioural therapy techniques (CBT) to challenge unhelpful thoughts like 'I can't cope', 'I'm a failure' and 'I'll never be happy again' (see 'Cognitive Behavioural Therapy' on page 85 onwards).

Additional very helpful information on cognitive behavioural therapy strategies for managing fatigue can be found in another book in the same *Overcoming* series as this one: *Overcoming Chronic Fatigue* by Mary Burgess and Trudie Chalder.

Tinnitus

Like long-term pain or fatigue, persisting tinnitus should first be investigated medically to check that there are no underlying health conditions that might be causing or contributing to it. This should include a hearing test as straining to hear things can cause the condition by itself. Correcting any hearing loss might therefore be an effective treatment in its own right. Once all medical assessments have been completed *tinnitus management strategies* might then be considered.

Understanding Tinnitus

In order to hear any noise our ears have to pick up sound waves and convert them into electrical impulses. These are then sent the brain and interpreted. Your brain, however, filters out huge amounts of background noise from your conscious awareness. This includes both external noises from your environment and internal ones from your body. Tinnitus occurs when this filter becomes too wide and it lets in some of these background noises into our awareness, e.g. whistling or hissing sounds. In other words, the threshold for filtering the impulses is lowered.

One of the key principles in the management of the condition is the understanding that stress, anxiety, low mood and fatigue can all widen the filter. Minimizing the effects these have on the filter therefore is one coping strategy. A second key principle is being aware that over time our thoughts and behaviours in relation to the condition can slowly change and add to the stress levels. This can involve us imperceptibly focusing our attention more and more on the unwanted sounds, avoiding more and more activities we previously found rewarding, and finding that the meaning the tinnitus has in our lives has become more and more negative. All of these can add fuel to the vicious cycle of tinnitus leading to stress, leading to more tinnitus, etc.

Managing Tinnitus

Some of the best ways to manage tinnitus include the following:

- Use relaxation techniques like anxiety management strategies, controlled breathing, physical exercise or meditation to minimize the stress–tinnitus vicious cycle (see 'What Can I Do to Manage the Physical Reactions?' on pages 92–94).

- Use sleep hygiene strategies to maximize sleep and minimize fatigue–tinnitus cycles (see 'Sleep' earlier in this book on pages 125–33). In particular, listening to quiet music or the radio in the background while getting off to sleep may help distract the mind from the tinnitus or from worrying thoughts that might be present.

- Distract yourself by undertaking and paying attention to enjoyable activities or those that give a sense of purpose and achievement, e.g. hobbies, DIY, voluntary work, DVDs, music.

- Use background music, the radio or other helpful noises to have sounds other than the tinnitus to focus on. Specialist devices called Environmental Sound Generators are also commercially available. These continually play soothing sounds (e.g. waves lapping or white noise) to have a different sound-focus.

- Use cognitive behavioural therapy techniques (CBT) to challenge unhelpful thoughts like 'I can't cope', 'I'm never going to get to sleep' and 'I'll never be happy again' (see 'Cognitive Behavioural Therapy' on page 85 onwards).

Tinnitus Retraining Therapy

Some people also find a specific treatment called Tinnitus Retraining (or Desensitization) Therapy helpful. This uses the idea that, over time, tinnitus noises can become processed in the parts of the brain that are also responsible for stress and emotional responses (the limbic system). This means that the sounds become harder and harder to ignore because they have more and more emotion attached to them, leading to the person becoming more and more conscious of them. It therefore uses a combination of getting used to background noises (sound therapy) alongside CBT techniques to help the brain get used to or habituate to the sounds so they are processed in the sub-conscious rather the conscious parts of our minds. This is a bit like us not being consciously aware of the background humming of a fridge because it is in our sub-conscious awareness until our attention is drawn to it. The therapy works on the basis that although the 'fridge' noise may be louder than normal it can still become a background, sub-conscious sound rather than a foreground, conscious one.

Dizziness and Sensitivity to Light or Noise

If you experience persistent problems with dizziness or sensitivity to light/noise you should in the first instance be assessed medically. This will ascertain whether there are any underlying health conditions that might be causing these problems and if any medical treatment for them is appropriate. Once this is completed the management strategies below might be considered.

Dizziness and sensitivity to light/noise, like other post-concussion type symptoms, can all be made worse by stress, depression, anxiety and similar factors. Indeed, these other factors, in and of themselves, can cause these difficulties even in the absence of a mild traumatic brain injury. Minimizing the vicious cycle therefore of dizziness or sensitivity to light/noise leading to increased stress/low mood, leading to further dizziness or sensitivity to light/noise can be an important management principle.

Physical exercise, relaxation techniques (see 'What Can I Do to Manage the Physical Reactions?' on pages 92–94), good sleep habits (see 'Sleep' on pages 125–33) and cognitive behavioural approaches (see 'Cognitive Behavioural Therapy' on pages 85 onwards) to examine and change the meaning these symptoms may have on your life can all be very helpful strategies to help reverse the vicious cycle. Carefully and systematically identifying the specific triggers for these problems and modifying behaviour accordingly may also help you gain more understanding and control in your life, further minimizing stress and the cycle.

As well as these general approaches there are some additional specific techniques for each of these problems.

Dizziness

Some forms of dizziness are due to changes in the ways that the ears, eyes and brain process information about the body's balance and spatial positions. Vestibular Rehabilitation Therapy is a set of individually tailored exercises that help retrain the brain to recognize, coordinate and interpret these signals more normally again. A physiotherapist or occupational therapist with training in this area is normally the professional who will undertake this kind of therapy. Once started the dizziness often gets a bit worse before improvements occur. It is, however, a very effective treatment for many and some regain complete normality balance through it.

Sensitivity to Noise

Some people with noise sensitivity find wearing earplugs, using hearing protection or listening to music in headphones helpful, particularly in environments that are noisy or problematic. Using earplugs or hearing protection, however, are not usually good long-term strategies as they can make the person even more sensitive to noise because of the increased contrast between long periods of quiet and normal sound levels. For many, *desensitization* is a more effective approach. This involves using a white-noise generator to slowly, systematically and in a very gradual way help the brain become accustomed to longer periods of louder noises. It uses the same principles as those used for anxiety-based avoidance behaviours (see 'Anxiety and Stress' on page 88 onwards).

Sensitivity to Light

Wearing good ultra-violet filter sunglasses or a wide-brimmed hat in situations where light sensitivity is at its worst can help many people with photophobia. Some find glasses with non-standard coloured lenses helpful. These are called *precision tinted lenses* and can be purchased from many good opticians.

SECTION 3

Information Sheets

The following are summaries of some of the key sections of this book in a format that is easy to scan or photocopy. They are designed as quick, user-friendly reminders of some of the self-help sections in this book. They contain the information that is most often needed by other people if they are going to be involved in helping you manage your post-concussion symptoms. They are not meant to be interventions in themselves but they may be useful in helping family, friends or other important people understand some of the issues and strategies relating to mild traumatic brain injury and post-concussion symptoms.

THE HUMAN BRAIN

The human brain is probably the most complicated thing in the universe. It weighs about 3lb (1.4 kg) and has the texture of toothpaste. It is made up of 50–100 billion nerve cells called neurons as well as 500–1,000 billion other cells. Neurons have a cell body with lots of branches coming off them called dendrites. They also have long tails called axons which are insulated by a sheath (myelin sheath). At the end of the axons are small branches called terminal branches. All of these branches form connections with other neurons making a vast number of connections throughout the brain.

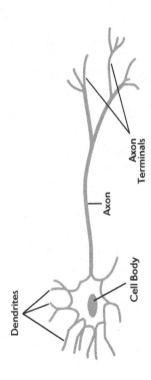

How Messages Are Sent

Messages are sent through these neurons by incredibly quick electrical charges which are relayed by incredibly quick chemical reactions. Different neurons can have different types of chemical transmitters that allow the messages to be passed from neuron to neuron. You may have heard of some of these – serotonin, noradrenaline, dopamine, etc. So throughout your life, even when you are sleeping, the brain is sending billions of messages through these neurons at extremely high speeds through vast numbers of chemical reactions. Messages are also sent to and from the brain by the neurons in the spinal cord in our backs and along the nerves in our bodies. These messages allow us to move our bodies and experience feeling. For example, when you decide to move your hand, messages from the brain travel down the neurons in your spinal cord through to the nerves in your hand which make the muscles move.

Different Parts of the Brain

On the surface of the brain the outer layer is about a quarter of an inch deep and is called the cortex. It is made up of a large concentration of neuron cell bodies, which gives it a grey-looking colour under the microscope. This is where the phrase 'using your grey matter' comes from. Below this area are a large number of neuron tails (axons). These act as connectors between different parts of the cortex a bit like a very complicated telephone wiring system. They are white in colour under the microscope.

Although the brain is extremely complicated we do know that different areas have different responsibilities. In most people, the left-hand side of the brain generally controls language, logical thinking, awareness of time and most things to do with written and spoken communication. The right-hand side of the brain is responsible for analysing visual information and for our experiences of three-dimensional space, artistic impression and 'intuition'. The main areas of the brain are also divided into different lobes which have different responsibilities although they all work in partnership with each other:

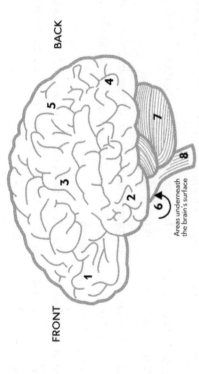

FRONT

BACK

Areas underneath the brain's surface

1. *Frontal Lobe* – The front part of the brain is responsible for planning, self-awareness, monitoring, coming up with ideas and putting ideas into action. These are often termed executive functions. There is an area on the left-hand side of the frontal area (Broca's area) that is responsible for finding the words and sentences we need when we speak or write.

2. *Temporal Lobe* – These are the areas on the lower sides of the brain. The left temporal

lobe normally controls the memory of verbal information, i.e. information that is written or spoken. The right temporal lobe is normally responsible for visual and spatial memory, i.e. information to do with vision and space. There is also an area towards the back of the left temporal area (Wernicke's area) that is responsible for understanding language.

3. *Sensory and Motor Strips* – There is a strip just behind the frontal lobe that controls the sending and receiving of messages about movements in your arms, shoulders, legs and other parts of your body. This is the motor strip. Immediately behind this is the sensory strip, which receives and sends messages of feeling from different parts of your body.

4. *Occipital Lobe* – At the back of the brain there is an area that controls the analysis of visual information sent from your eyes to the brain.

5. *Parietal Lobe* – The area on the upper side of the brain behind the sensory strip is called the parietal lobe. The right parietal lobe processes information to do with space and the awareness of your body movements.

6. *Sub-cortical areas* – These are the areas of the brain underneath the cortical area. They are involved with controlling feelings, emotions, pain, temperature, movement and general levels of alertness.

7. *Cerebellum* – This large part of the brain at the back controls the coordination of movements that we decide to make.

8. *Brain Stem* – This area of the brain just above the top of the spinal cord controls our basic life-support systems like breathing, swallowing and how conscious we are.

Dr Nigel King,

Consultant Clinical Neuropsychologist

TRAUMATIC BRAIN INJURY

One of the most important things to know about traumatic brain injury is that all head injuries are different and each person's response to a head injury is different. There is therefore no such thing as a 'typical head injury'.

The terms 'traumatic brain injury' and 'head injury' are often used to describe exactly the same thing and they cover a very broad range of injuries. They include mild traumatic brain injury, which normally involves no measurable brain damage and complete recovery within a few days, through to extremely severe brain damage resulting in permanent coma or death. Some of the best ways to measure the severity of a head injury include:

1. the length of any unconsciousness associated with the injury;
2. the period of time between suffering the injury and regaining moment-by-moment memory for events – post traumatic amnesia;
3. the depth of any changes in consciousness immediately after the injury. This is often measured by the Glasgow Coma Scale (GCS) score, which runs from 3 (the most deeply unconscious you can be) to 15 (full consciousness and full orientation);

4. the results of any neurological investigations that may have been necessary, e.g. CT or MRI brain scans (these, however, are not necessary after most mild head injuries).

Generally speaking the longer the period of unconsciousness, the greater the depth of unconsciousness; and the longer the length of post-traumatic amnesia the more severe the head injury is likely to be.

Severity of Head Injury

A very crude assessment of severity of head injury would be:

- *'Mild or moderate head injury'* when post-traumatic amnesia is less than twenty-four hours.

- *'Severe head injury'* when post-traumatic amnesia is between one to seven days.

- *'Very severe head injury'* when post-traumatic amnesia is more than seven days.

It should be recognized, however, that these are very much 'rough rule of thumb' indicators of injury severity and that there are huge variations in outcome even within these categories.

Damage to the Brain after Severe and Very Severe Injuries

After a severe or very severe head injury damage to the brain can occur due to i) the brain being bruised (contusion), ii) nerve cells (neurons) being damaged or destroyed, iii) connections between nerve cells being damaged and iv) the veins and arteries which provide blood to the brain being torn. The latter can lead to bleeding (haemorrhage) and lack of oxygen to the brain causing damage or death of nerve cells. As a result the messages that are sent through these damaged areas are disrupted. This type of damage is called 'primary damage'. There can also be 'secondary damage' if the head injury causes swelling in the brain, brain infection or not enough oxygen to get to the brain because of breathing difficulties or very low blood pressure.

Often in a severe head injury the front of the brain (frontal lobes) and lower sides of the brain (temporal lobes) are the areas that receive the most damage. This is because there are sharp parts of the skull that stick out here and during a severe head injury the brain moves within the skull causing damage in these areas. There is also often damage to the nerve cell tails (axons) over lots of areas of the brain due to the brain stretching or rubbing against itself (diffuse axonal shearing).

Improvement after Head Injury

Even though there is no such thing as a 'typical' head injury, after very severe head injuries there is always *some degree* of natural healing of the brain. Generally most recovery takes place over the first one to two years. The improvements then tend to slow down and level out. Small amounts of natural recovery can continue for a long time afterwards, although these tend to be much smaller improvements compared with those that occur in the first year or two. Improvements in how a person copes with everyday life, however, can go on indefinitely as they learn to adapt and find ways around the difficulties that arise. It is impossible to say early on after a very severe head injury how much natural improvement is likely to occur and whether the person will get back to 99 per cent of their original mental capacity or 85 per cent or 50 per cent, etc. This becomes clearer as time goes on. Some permanent reduction in mental ability, however, is usual after a very severe head injury.

The natural recovery after severe head injury is not fully understood, but it probably involves:

1. the chemicals which transmit the electrical message in the brain cells (neurons) settling down and regaining some of their original efficiency;

2. some of the damaged neurons or their connections repairing themselves;

3. the swelling and bruising in the brain reducing causing the neurons in these areas to function more efficiently.

It may possibly also involve undamaged areas of the brain taking on some of the responsibilities that damaged areas used to do (neuroplasticity). However, not everyone agrees about how much this can occur.

Cognitive Rehabilitation

As well as the natural recovery of the brain following a head injury, significant improvements in a person's day-to-day life can occur as a result of *cognitive rehabilitation*. This involves providing detailed information about head injury to the person and their family or friends, assessing the person's thinking skills to identify their specific strengths and weaknesses and finding practical ways to solve the problems that the brain injury causes, e.g. using a diary to help memory and planning problems. It can also include relearning specific skills a person needs for everyday life. This not only helps the person relearn the skills they need but may also help stimulate the areas of the brain responsible for these things, therefore aiding its natural recovery.

Dr Nigel King,
Consultant Clinical Neuropsychologist

MILD TRAUMATIC BRAIN INJURY AND PROLONGED POST CONCUSSION-TYPE SYMPTOMS

Definition

Some of the best ways to measure the severity of a traumatic brain injury include:

1. the length of any unconsciousness associated with the injury;

2. the period of time between suffering the injury and regaining moment-by-moment memory for events – post-traumatic amnesia;

3. the depth of any changes in consciousness immediately after the injury. This is often measured by the Glasgow Coma Scale (GCS) score, which runs from 3 (the most deeply unconscious you can be) to 15 (full consciousness and orientation).

4. the results of any neurological investigations that may have been necessary, e.g. CT or MRI brain scans (these, however, are not necessary after most mild head injuries).

A mild traumatic brain injury (MTBI) or mild head injury (MHI) is defined as one resulting in unconsciousness of less than fifteen minutes, post-traumatic amnesia of less than twenty-four hours, an initial GCS of 13–15 and no evidence of significant brain injury with neurological investigations.

Post-concussion Symptoms

Post-concussion symptoms (PCS) are a range of difficulties that often occur as a result of a mild traumatic brain injury. They include headaches, dizziness, fatigue, irritability, sleep disturbance, reduced day-to-day memory, poor concentration, taking longer to think, depression, anxiety, tinnitus, blurred or double vision, sensitivity to light or noise, frustration, nausea, restlessness and sensitivity to alcohol. For the vast majority these symptoms completely resolve over the first few weeks or months.

Persisting Symptoms

Unfortunately a minority of patients suffer from persisting or long-term PCS. This will often mean that the term 'mild traumatic brain injury' does not in any way adequately describe the consequences of the injury as ongoing PCS can be very disabling indeed and affect almost all aspects of life. Such difficulties are frequently called a 'hidden disability' as the person usually looks fine and in a range of situations may show no obvious effects of the injury.

Different Opinions

Post-concussion type symptoms are not very specific and nearly all of them can be caused by things completely unrelated to a mild traumatic brain injury. These include: chronic pain, stress, low mood, reduced quality or quantity of sleep, the emotional consequences of a psychological trauma (post-traumatic stress), physical or cognitive symptoms caused by emotional disturbances (somatoform problems), anxiety and chronic fatigue problems. Unfortunately some of these factors are often present after a MTBI or can develop as a response to the large increases in effort that are needed to try to cope with PCS.

Some clinicians are of the opinion that early on PCS are caused by the MTBI itself but that long term post-concussion-type symptoms are always due to the development of non-head injury factors over time. In other words, the symptoms may not change as time goes on but the causes of them do. Other clinicians say that persisting PCS are always caused by the mild traumatic brain injury itself – possibly because they are not aware of the other factors that cause the same difficulties, e.g. stress causing day-to-day memory problems, pain causing poor concentration, anxiety causing blurred vision, etc. Still others will be open-minded to the possibility that both head injury and non-head injury factors (and the interactions between both factors) can be responsible for prolonged symptoms.

Vicious Cycles

As you can see a person may get very different opinions from clinicians about their difficulties after a MTBI. What we do know is that age (e.g. being over forty) and gender (being female) can increase the likelihood of experiencing prolonged post-concussion-type symptoms. We also know that any direct effects of a mild traumatic brain injury improve over time. The natural healing processes that occur in the brain, however, can be very slow and in some cases maximum brain injury recovery may take one to two years.

While head injury factors will reduce over time, non-head injury factors may well increase – especially if the person struggles to understand and manage their PCS. Vicious cycles between different symptoms, however, often develop as time goes on, regardless of the cause of PCS. These significantly add to the difficulties experienced, e.g. reduced concentration leading to increased stress, causing further concentration difficulties, causing more stress, etc. Natural characteristics like perfectionistic tendencies, 'all-or-nothing' approaches to dealing with problems or a strong desire to control things may also add to the difficulties in managing persisting PCS.

What Helps?

A very useful first thing that can help someone suffering from prolonged post-concussion-type symptoms is to make a list of all the head injury and non-head injury factors that might possibly be causing their symptoms. The second thing may then be to decide which symptoms could be causing vicious cycles of problems as there are often many of these with prolonged PCS. A third thing may then be to explore if the difficulties have affected the way the person feels, thinks and behaves, and any vicious cycles that may have developed in these areas.

A clinician will sometimes help this process and may summarize these factors in a box diagram to create an individualized explanation of the specific difficulties and their causes for the person. This then means that one 'box' can be tackled at a time and vicious cycles can be reduced and 'virtuous cycles' increased. By slowing tackling the difficulties 'one box at a time' substantial improvements can be made in both reducing PCS and effectively managing any that remain. The good news is that there are many proven ways of tackling the individual 'boxes', e.g. stress may be helped by stress-management training taken from mental health resources; day-to-day memory problems may be helped by cognitive rehabilitation strategies taken from severe brain injury resources; unhelpful feelings/thoughts/behaviour may be reduced by specific forms of psychological interventions such as cognitive behavioural therapy.

Remember: *'Knowledge is power' and having an individualized explanation for your PCS may be the important first step to finding solutions to your problems.*

Dr Nigel King,

Consultant Clinical Neuropsychologist

REDUCED THINKING STAMINA

Your thinking stamina can be reduced for many different reasons (e.g. post-concussion symptoms, stress, low mood, pain, brain injury). If this happens you may find that you cope with the demands of everyday life less well and you need to pace yourself more carefully in managing your work and daily activities.

A Possible Cause

Reduced thinking stamina can occur because the information processing capacity of the brain is lowered. This means that the person is less able to process as *much* information as before or as *quickly* as before. In other words, the brain is more easily overloaded.

Symptoms You May Notice

Slowness – as information has to be taken on board in smaller amounts.

Distractibility – as it takes more effort to continue concentrating on an activity.

Forgetfulness – as less information can be stored at any one time.

Fatigue – as the brain has to work harder to process information.

Irritability – as the mind is under more stress.

Common Problems

Things that can be difficult during this time are:

1. activities that require multi-tasking or long periods of concentration, e.g. cooking a meal from scratch, reading a book, listening to a lecture or writing a report;

2. activities where more than one person is talking, e.g. meetings or social occasions;

3. activities where a lot of people are around you, e.g. shopping, working in a shared office or having young children wanting attention;

4. non-routine tasks, e.g. entertaining visitors or visiting unfamiliar places;

5. working fast to meet a deadline.

What Helps?

Things which can help include:

1. rearranging working environments to minimize background noise, 'busyness', unexpected events, time pressures and distractions, e.g. radio, computer, mobile phone or television;

2. breaking activities down into small sections with lots of small breaks in between, i.e. pacing tasks more;

3. doing *routine and familiar* tasks when fatigue and concentration are 'at their worst', e.g. at the end of an afternoon or end of a week;

4. doing *new and unfamiliar* tasks when you are 'at your best', e.g. in the morning or at the beginning of a week;

5. always using a diary to plan the day, pace yourself and remind yourself of things you need to do, e.g. appointments;

6. cutting down on non-essential activity – this may involve learning to say 'No' to things more: do not feel guilty about this;

7. taking many small breaks *before* impairments become apparent rather than 'pushing on' until forced to take a break due to 'cognitive overload';

8. returning to pre-injury activities very gradually and systematically over time.

9. identifying specific times or specific types of activity where fatigue, irritability, anxiety or frustration occur and making appropriate changes in these areas;

10. allowing extra time for tasks where multi-tasking is required.

Remember: *Pacing yourself, taking lots of small breaks during activities and not overstretching yourself are often the keys to effectively managing reduced thinking stamina.*

Dr Nigel King,

Consultant Clinical Neuropsychologist

MEMORY

There are many different reasons why someone may have problems with their memory (e.g. post-concussion symptoms, stress, low mood, pain, brain injury). These problems generally occur for 'short-term' or day-to-day memory because older memories are usually much better established. In other words, it is new information that is often harder to remember and learn.

The Remembering Process

The process of remembering involves three different stages:

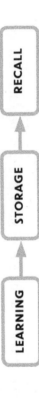

1. *Learning* – When you first concentrate on something.
2. *Storage* – The things you have learned are stored.
3. *Recall* – Getting information you have learnt to hand when you need it.

Memory is a bit like a filing cabinet where memories are organized in an efficient filing system, making it easy to get information out when you want to remember it. There are many different files or types of memory: memory for faces, memory for events, memory for facts, memory for verbal information, memory for visual or spatial information, memory for physical acts and memory for the things we do on 'autopilot' because we have done them many times before. If any of these files are working less efficiently, memory lapses can occur i.e. the filing system is less effective or slowed down. Even if the information gets into the filing system and is stored, the system may be disorganized so the person gets muddled or confused. The memory can be affected because some of the files are less efficient at storing information (storage) or because the retrieval of information from the files is less efficient (recall).

Common Memory Problems

- Forgetting names, times, appointments, places, routes, phone numbers.
- Forgetting your train of thought, i.e. getting verbal blanks.
- Having words on the tip of your tongue and not being able to find the right words.

Things to Bear in Mind

1. Memory is not like a muscle and cannot be made better by doing exercises. Instead it is better to adapt to your changed memory and use strategies that can help overcome any difficulties, e.g. use a diary to write down appointments or write notes to remind you what you need to do.

2. Remember that nobody's memory is perfect. Therefore, try to avoid saying things like 'I'm stupid, I'm always forgetting things' as this may make you feel your memory is worse than it actually is.

3. Memory can be made worse by poor concentration so try not to do too many things at once. Your memory can also be affected by increases in anxiety, tiredness, irritability, frustration and stress, so try to keep these at manageable levels.

4. Try to be well organized in your everyday life, e.g. do certain things at certain times, have set routines and always leave things that you use a lot in their right place.

Helping Your Memory

The best way of helping difficulties with your memory is usually to accept the difficulties and adopt strategies to help get around the problems. It is then a matter of finding which strategy is most suited to your needs and lifestyle and being disciplined about using it. At first, while you are getting used to a new strategy, you may find things get worse before they get better. This is normal and some perseverance is usually necessary for at least a few weeks. Here is a list of some of the strategies that may be useful.

Using a Diary, Electronic Reminders (e.g. Mobile Phone) or Notebook

The most helpful memory strategy is often to use a diary, electronic reminder (e.g. mobile phone) or notebook in a very systematic way. It is most effective when used to plan and look ahead to things you need to do in the near future or to record important information you need to remember. The size and type of diary or reminder does not really matter but it is a good idea to get in the habit of carrying it around with you all the time in your pocket or handbag. This way you will always have it to hand when you need to write something down or check it. It is often a good idea to attach a pen or pencil to the diary or notebook so you always have something with which to write.

How to Use Your Diary, Electronic Reminder or Notebook

Have a set time in the day when you write down your plans for the day or put in any future information in your diary, notebook, mobile phone etc. Generally the best times are first thing in the morning or last thing at night. Try to get into the habit of checking your diary or device at regular intervals throughout the day, e.g. every hour or two.

What to Put in It:

Fill in the front pages with information such as names, phone numbers and addresses.

1. Every day put in appointments (e.g. doctor's appointments) including names, times, places and anything else you need to remember about the appointment (e.g. things you need to ask about).

2. Include things you need to know about the day (e.g. partner will be late in and where they are).

3. Include tasks that need to be done that day (e.g. pick cousin up from station).

4. Include things people have told you or you need to tell them (e.g. ask neighbour to return lawnmower).

As you complete tasks and do things it is a good idea to cross them out or tick them off.

Other Memory Strategies

Other memory aids which can help are:

1. being as organized as possible in your everyday life, e.g. doing certain things at set times and have set routines;

2. writing down information on sticky notes and sticking them in places where you will need to remember the information;

3. using alarms on watches, mobile phones or clocks to remind you to do things like take medication or look at your diary/reminder;

4. using a mobile phone, computer or electronic organizer and setting reminders that prompt you to do things;

5. using a tape recorder/Dictaphone to help you remember things (e.g. when attending a meeting/lecture);

6. asking a friend or relative to remind you to do things;

7. using a white board, notice board or calendar to quickly and regularly remind you of information (e.g. to buy someone's birthday present);

8. using satnav devices to find your way to new or unfamiliar places;

9. developing a tidy living and working environment where belongings are kept in the same, intuitively obvious, places and can easily be found; this helps to minimize demand on memory and problem-solving skills and make maximum use of non-conscious memory capacity;

10. taking pictures on a mobile phone as a reminder of significant things done previously in the day/week/month, etc.;

11. systematically using written or photo journals for episodic memory deficits (memory for personal events).

12. systematizing storage of household items with explicit labelling (e.g. colour coding);

13. using 'errorless learning' when learning new skills to minimize the need to 'unlearn' mistakes, i.e. getting others to prompt and cue you in such a way that no errors are made during a training process.

Mental Strategies

Some people also find mental memory strategies helpful. It should be noted that the degree of mental effort required for such 'internal' memory strategies often exceeds their usefulness for people with memory impairments. They can be useful, however, for specific tasks like remembering names of people or studying for an exam where external strategies are inappropriate. These are some of the most effective ones:

1. Repetition can help you to remember. Going over the information in your mind regularly can reinforce and help the learning stage of the memory process. You might also ask people to repeat information to help you remember what they have said.

2. Associations can help when you need to remember specific information e.g. to remember the name Bob Fish, you might think of a person bobbing up and down with a fish on their head.

3. Chunking information together can help reduce the memory load e.g. to remember a telephone number such as 01799486358, chunk the numbers together: 01-799-48-63-58.

4. Either visualizing or verbalizing what you have to remember can help, e.g. when trying to find your way in an unfamiliar place visualize landmarks to help you on your way back, or when remembering a route from a map talk through instructions of how to get to your destination.

Dr Nigel King,
Consultant Clinical Neuropsychologist

EXECUTIVE FUNCTIONING

In a company the executive or boss has an important job. The executive has to: keep check on how the company is doing; plan for the future; put into practice different ways of working; and change how the company does things when circumstances change. The executive often has to stand back from the company and be flexible and creative.

The 'executive functioning' of the brain does a similar job to the boss in a company. Problems in this area of thinking can affect nearly all aspects of thinking and acting and can show up in many different ways. The most common ways are:

1. *Coming up with ideas or intentions*

   People can find it difficult to think of things they would like to do. They can appear to have little energy, be less motivated or to have lost their 'get up and go'. Sometimes it seems like their 'spark' has gone. These problems can be mistaken for laziness or apathy.

2. *Starting and stopping movements or ideas*

   Moving parts of the body in particular ways may be difficult to get started. Sometimes movements can be more difficult to stop once they have got going. This can also happen when speaking or thinking. People can have problems in coming up with words and ideas or putting ideas into action. Once started, these may then be repeated when they would usually have stopped. This difficulty in stopping movements, words or thoughts is called 'perseveration'.

3. *Concrete thinking*

People may find it difficult to be flexible with thoughts or ideas. They can appear rigid or unable to 'let go' of fixed ideas. They can find it difficult to think in general or abstract ways, and can have problems in understanding jokes and irony, or in answering open-ended questions, e.g. 'What would you like to do today?' Problems in putting themselves in the other person's shoes may also be present. Such problems can be mistaken for selfishness or awkwardness.

4. *Planning*

Working out what steps are needed to put ideas into action can be difficult. People can seem to never get round to putting their ideas into practice or doing things they say they will do. Breaking tasks down into small steps can be very difficult. Problems in thinking through actions before doing them may also be present and show up as impulsivity. This can be mistaken for carelessness.

5. *Checking*

Problems in 'standing back' and checking things out can occur. People can appear slapdash.

6. *Responding to social signals*

People can have problems in learning through the advice and feedback of people around them. When with others the less obvious signals that are used in conversations like suggestions, body language and smiles can be particularly difficult for people to notice or use. As a consequence social rules may be broken more often, e.g. over-familiarity with strangers may occur because the rule about getting to know people slowly is not used or someone might be very talkative because the rule about taking turns in conversation is not followed. The person may also have less insight and awareness of problems and difficulties they might have. They may therefore struggle to recognize when difficulties arise or accept help with them.

People with executive difficulties sometimes have particular patterns of problems. Some can tend to have most problems in acting without thinking, following social rules and interpreting words and sentences in too many different ways. Others can tend to have problems getting themselves going, taking rules and regulations too seriously, and interpreting words and sentences in very literal ways, e.g. having difficulties in understanding figures of speech and proverbs. These patterns of problems are like the opposite sides of the same coin when it comes to executive functioning.

Practical things that may help with executive problems are:

1. Breaking tasks down into small, logical steps. This can help provide the structure and planning with which the person may have problems. An example might be 'to make the sandwich you must i) get the bread, ii) find a knife, butter and jam, iii) butter the bread, iv) spread jam on one of the slices and v) put the bread together'.

2. Using a diary to write down a structure and routine for each day and week. The diary should be carried and used at all times so that it becomes a habit to use it. This can help plan *what* to do each day, *when* to do it and *how* to do it. A diary is particularly important when someone has memory problems as well as executive ones.

3. Getting those who know the person well to ask multiple-choice questions rather than open-ended ones. An example might be 'Would you rather go to the shops or swimming tomorrow?' rather than 'What would you like to do tomorrow?' This can make it easier to make a decision.

4. Getting those who know the person well to tell them or signal to them when they are

breaking social rules, e.g. when they need to stop talking because someone else is ready to say something. This can give valuable feedback about social rules. It *must only* be done when the person and others agree to it and when one specific social rule for feedback has been agreed upon.

5. Using a watch with an alarm, mobile phone 'alarm/reminder' function or a paging device as a cue to look at a diary and initiate particular tasks.

6. Using notes, calendars and lists as external cues to help initiate tasks.

7. Undertaking problem-solving skills training to help develop an explicit and systematic approach to solving difficulties, e.g. i) defining the problem to be overcome; ii) generating different strategies to overcome the problem; iii) highlighting the pros and cons of each strategy; iv) deciding the best strategy based on the pros and cons; v) implementing the strategy; and vi) evaluating the outcome.

8. Using an alarmed stopwatch/mobile phone to help monitor the amount of time taken on given tasks to help planning and time-judgement impairments.

9. Talking to oneself about a task (verbal mediation) to help overcome initiation problems and to be reminded of any self statements that help social awareness.

10. Introducing repeated routines/cycles to reduce unnecessary decision-making (e.g. weekly menus, shopping lists, set times for visiting the gym, etc.).

Remember: *Structure and routine can be the keys to helping with executive problems.*

Dr Nigel King,
Consultant Clinical Neuropsychologist

COGNITIVE REHABILITATION

In addition to the specific strategies that can help common thinking problems, general cognitive rehabilitation principles can also be very important in achieving the best possible coping skills. Because the brain is not like a muscle, exercising a particular part of it using 'brain training' mental exercises usually makes very little difference to a person's real-life functioning. They are likely to improve their performance on the specific exercise being undertaken but are unlikely to gain any improved cognitive ability. Having said this, it is important to maintain a reasonable level of mental stimulation to keep mental health optimal but without 'overdoing it', which can lead to fatigue, irritability, stress or depression. The main focus in cognitive rehabilitation therefore is in developing a detailed understanding of the person's individual strengths and weaknesses in their thinking skills and creatively finding alternative practical ways of achieving the best day-to-day functioning.

Cognitive Rehabilitation Strategies

There are three important principles that substantially help to achieve optimal cognitive rehabilitation.

1. *Reducing 'mental load'*

   A large number of factors can cause the brain to work on 'reduced capacity'. These include post-concussion symptoms, stress, pain, anxiety, fatigue and brain injury. This is like a car running on three cylinders instead of four. In other words, the brain is constantly working harder than it would normally do. Everyday tasks therefore use up much more mental energy than before. This means that it is much easier to become mentally 'overloaded'. The most effective way of managing this problem is by reducing the 'mental load' on the brain. This can be done by:

   a) taking lots of small breaks during the day;
   b) using routines and familiar or 'autopilot' tasks as much as possible;
   c) undertaking small, achievable goals one at a time rather than altogether;
   d) maintaining a good balance between resting and mental stimulation;

e) developing daily and weekly routines that involve meaningful daytime activities, e.g. voluntary work;

f) using practical 'compensatory' strategies to get around cognitive difficulties, e.g. using a diary for day-to-day memory difficulties;

g) returning to activities slowly and in small steps (progressing to each new step only when the previous step has been achieved);

h) minimizing self-criticism and self-blame regarding any difficulties caused by the mild traumatic brain injury;

i) avoiding taking on too many activities and responsibilities at any one time (this may involve learning to say 'No' more effectively).

2. *Mood management*

Emotional reactions like frustration, anger, irritability, loss of confidence, stress, anxiety and depression are very normal when managing cognitive difficulties. These emotional reactions, however, can make cognitive difficulties worse. While this is not physically harmful it can lead to a vicious cycle where cognitive difficulties are made worse by emotional reactions, which then lead to greater cognitive difficulties etc. Alongside this, it is important to know that the process of adjusting to such problems often involves difficult emotions and is a slow process. Some people view it as a kind of emotional journey involving challenges along the way but with positive emotional growth occurring as understanding, insight and realistic hope are developed. For some this involves accepting at least part of themselves as being a 'new person'. This means that while they are the same person as before, they learn to accept some different characteristics in their make-up.

3. *Acceptance*

Two key elements of cognitive rehabilitation are:

a) understanding and accepting limitations;
b) finding practical ways to get around these difficulties.

Finding practical solutions to problems is often called 'compensation' and is far more effective than trying to restore lost thinking skills through mental exercises. Often people can push themselves to exhaustion in order to try to 'get back to normal' as soon as possible. This, however, often feels like 'wearing a mask' or 'putting on a brave face' when the person is actually struggling inside. It can be a relief to acknowledge this and 'take off the mask' to begin adjusting to things more openly.

This can sometimes be slowed down by the natural process of 'denial', which can help protect a person from having to work through difficult issues until they are ready to do so. It often takes some time to fully understand, accept and adjust to limitations and being able to talk openly with someone about these things can help enormously. It can also be very beneficial for the person to have realistic (but supportive) feedback about their strengths and weaknesses from those close to them.

Remember: *Cognitive rehabilitation is about: i) understanding strengths and weaknesses; ii) finding practical solutions to problems; iii) positively adjusting to new aspects of life. The challenges are often both mental and emotional but offer the prospect of positive personal growth and insight along the way.*

Dr Nigel King,
Consultant Clinical Neuropsychologist

COGNITIVE REHABILITATION STRATEGIES

The following is a list of some of the most commonly used cognitive rehabilitation strategies. Strategies should also be developed individually by you to creatively find potential ways to manage your own specific cognitive strengths and weaknesses.

The keys to employing any strategy effectively are:

1. understanding your own individual cognitive strengths and weaknesses;

2. identifying only one new strategy to try at any one time and being certain that this is the one *you* want as *your* goal;

3. acknowledging that until a new strategy has become a habit, it can take some effort to keep going with it. Usually after 4–8 weeks of consistent practice it will become a routine part of your daily life. If you are able to 'attach' the new strategy to a habit or routine you already have in place this can make it easier to learn. When you are able to use a strategy almost on 'autopilot' it will then be an effective technique.

General Cognitive Strategies

- *Developing habits, routines and 'autopilot' procedures* to: i) maximize the use of automatic, non-conscious memory functions; ii) provide structure; and iii) minimize mental load.

- *Developing a tidy living and working environment* where belongings are kept in the same, intuitively obvious, places and can easily be found. This helps to minimize demand on memory and problem-solving skills and make maximum use of non-conscious memory capacity.

- *Taking many small breaks when impairments become apparent* rather than 'pushing on' until forced to take a break due to 'cognitive overload'.

- *Rearranging working environments* to minimize background noise, 'busyness', unexpected events and time pressures. This helps to reduce restrictions arising from attentional deficits, slow speed of information processing and less flexible thinking.

- *Graduated return to pre-injury activities and minimization of non-essential activity* to reduce cognitive overload and fatigue. This maximizes the chances of successful completion of activities.

- *Identifying specific times or specific types of activity where fatigue, irritability, anxiety or frustration occur and making appropriate changes in these areas.*

- *Allowing extra time for tasks where judgement of time or speed of information processing is reduced.*

- *Using a diary, electronic diary or 'diary' function on a mobile phone systematically as i) a reminder of things to remember, ii) a means of structuring time, iii) a means of orientating to place and time, iv) an aid to overcoming problems initiating a task (getting started), or v) a reminder of key messages and conclusions from consultations/meetings.*

Strategies for Managing Memory

- *Using a Dictaphone/tape recorder to record meetings, lectures, etc. as a reminder of things to remember.*

- *Using a watch with an alarm, mobile phone 'alarm/reminder' function or a paging device as a cue to look at a diary or to perform particular tasks. (This may also help you get started on the task if you have difficulties with initiation).*

- *Using satnav devices* to overcome route-finding memory difficulties.

- *Taking pictures on a mobile phone* as a reminder of significant things done previously in the day/week/month, etc.

- *Systematically using written or photo journals* for episodic memory deficits (i.e. memory for events).

- *Using notes, calendars and lists* as external cues and reminders. These may also help problems with initiating tasks.

- *Introducing a notice board or white board* in a prominent place in the home to be regularly prompted about specific actions, as well as daily/weekly schedules.

- *Systematizing storage of household items with explicit labelling* (e.g. colour coding) (Such strategies are especially important for safety of toxic substances for people with visual perception difficulties).

- *Using errorless learning* when learning new skills to minimize the need to 'unlearn' mistakes, i.e. getting others to prompt and cue you in such a way that no errors are made during a training process.

- *Developing internal memory strategies* via repetition, association, chunking, verbalization of visual material or maximizing the relevance and depth of understanding of material. It should be noted, however, that the degree of mental effort required for such 'internal' memory strategies often exceeds their usefulness for people with memory and executive impairments. They can, however, be useful for specific tasks like remembering names of people or studying for an exam where external strategies are inappropriate.

Strategies for Executive Difficulties

- *Providing problem-solving skills training* to help develop an explicit and systematic approach to solving difficulties, e.g. i) defining the problem to be overcome; ii) generating different strategies to overcome the problem; iii) highlighting the pros and cons of each strategy; iv) deciding the best strategy based on the pros and cons; v) implementing the strategy; and vi) evaluating the outcome.

- *Using an alarmed stopwatch/mobile phone* to help monitor the amount of time taken on tasks to help planning and time-judgement impairments.

- *Talking to yourself about a task (verbal mediation)* to help overcome initiation problems and to be reminded of any self statements that help your social awareness.

- *Breaking tasks down into small, 'bite-sized' steps with written instructions* to reduce problems from planning deficits.

- *Introducing repeated routines/cycles* to reduce unnecessary decision-making (e.g. weekly menus, shopping lists, set times for visiting the gym, etc.).

Strategies for Behavioural Management

- *Identifying a small range of people to provide behavioural feedback* to help modify inappropriate social behaviours. This should be done with careful and sensitive collaboration between you and those providing the feedback. (It is important to stress that the feedback should be immediate, concrete, supportive and constructive, and aimed at very specific behaviours only).

- *Using a handheld counter* to aid the self-monitoring of specified inappropriate social behaviours.

- *Using video feedback* to improve insight into specific inappropriate behaviours.

As people may be surprised or upset by being confronted with inappropriate behaviours, strategies should always be: i) discussed and negotiated carefully with the person; ii) undertaken in a controlled and supportive atmosphere; and iii) conducted with sufficient time allocated for debriefing immediately afterwards.

Strategies for Social Skills

- *Learn conversation skills* for slowing, pacing and allowing 'thinking time' during interactions to help minimize word-finding, sentence-construction and concentration difficulties in conversation.

- *Learn social skills* so that you are comfortable asking for things to be repeated during conversation when attention, memory or language deficits have caused you to lose track.

- *Encourage others to use short sentences and simpler words* and to allow enough time for you to reply to questions when word-finding, attentional, receptive language or expressive language impairments are present.

- *Encourage those close to you to use closed, multiple-choice-type questions* rather than open-ended questions where decision making and initiation of ideas are impaired.

Remember: *Strategies will only become useful once they become a habit and part of your daily routine. Quite a lot of effort and practice will be needed for this to happen, but once it does the strategies will be 'worth their weight in gold'.*

Dr Nigel King,
Consultant Clinical Neuropsychologist

Source: Adapted from N. S. King and A. Tyerman, 'The neuropsychological presentation and treatment of traumatic brain injury', in J. M. Gurd, U. Kischka and J. C. Marshall (eds), *The Handbook of Clinical Neuropsychology*, Oxford: Oxford University Press, 2010. Reprinted with permission.

SECTION 4

Conclusions and 'Take Home Messages'

There are eight key 'take home messages' that I hope you have taken from this book. They are exactly the same as those mentioned at the beginning. So if you remember them just skip to the 'Final Word'!

1. *The Brain Is Incredibly Complicated*

   The brain is the most complicated thing in the universe and although we know a great deal about how it works there is still a huge amount that we do not understand about it.

2. *Mild Traumatic Brain Injury Does Not Always Have 'Mild' Consequences*

   If you have suffered a mild traumatic brain injury and are experiencing ongoing post-concussion symptoms then the term 'mild' is likely to be a very inaccurate way of describing your problems. Your symptoms may well affect many areas of your life and may severely limit what you are able to do.

3. *Same Symptoms, Different Causes and Different Explanations*

Post-concussion symptoms and many problems after mild traumatic brain injury can be identical to those caused by other factors – including stress, pain, physical difficulties, sleep disturbance, emotional difficulties and severe brain injury. This may make it very difficult to understand your problems. This is made worse by the differing explanations you may receive from different clinicians. Some may tell you that your ongoing problems are caused by your brain injury. Others may say they are caused by emotional and psychological factors. Still others may believe that both brain injury and emotional factors are at work. These opinions may well be stated very confidently even though they are very different! Clearly this will not help you to understand your problems. In many ways, however, the more that your difficulties are actually caused by non-brain injury factors the better it is. This is because there will be a greater chance that they may be fully overcome.

4. *Stand Back from Your Problems to 'See the Wood for the Trees'*

Regardless of the extent to which your symptoms are caused by brain injury or non-brain injury factors, the best place to start to understand them is to write a list of all the different things that might contribute to your current symptoms. This will help start the process of standing back from your problems to 'see the wood from the trees' and to gain a bird's-eye view of your difficulties.

The list might include thinking difficulties such as: reduced multi-tasking abilities; mental fatigue; poor concentration; slower thinking speed; short-term memory deficits; reduced mental stamina; troubles with planning; or difficulties with problem solving. They might also include emotional difficulties such as: post-traumatic stress; anxieties surrounding a compensation claim or other legal proceedings; worries about family or work tasks; perfectionism; anger or irritability; low mood; driving anxiety; or concerns about the head injury itself. Additional difficulties may involve physical problems. These might include: poorer sleep; headaches; tiredness; pain; sensitivity to light or noise; dizziness; or tinnitus.

5. *Create a Full Personalized Explanation of Your Specific Problems*

A vital step may then be to create a full, personalized explanation of your specific problems. Often this will be in the form of a 'Box Diagram' for your own condition. This will help highlight what vicious cycles have developed over time and which ones are maintaining your symptoms or making them worse.

This can be the most important step in overcoming PCS as 'knowledge is power' when it comes to managing MTBI.

6. *Cognitive Behavioural and Cognitive Rehabilitation Strategies*

The most effective strategies for tackling each of the 'boxes' will probably come from cognitive rehabilitation or cognitive behavioural therapy (CBT) approaches. The cognitive rehabilitation strategies that work best are the 'external' ones rather than 'brain training' exercises. These involve finding practical ways to get around the different types of thinking difficulties you may have. The key principles involved are:

a) Understanding your own individual cognitive strengths and weaknesses.

b) Identifying only one new strategy to try at any one time and being certain that this is the one *you* want as *your* goal.

c) Acknowledging that until a new strategy has become a habit, it can take some effort to keep going with it. Usually after 4–8 weeks of consistent practice it will become a routine part of your daily life.

The cognitive behavioural approaches involve understanding the powerful idea that feelings, thoughts, actions and bodily sensations do not just interact with each other in one direction – they interact in a combination of all directions. CBT then involves identifying vicious cycles caused by these different factors 'playing off each other' and using techniques to reverse them so they become 'virtuous cycles'.

7. *Do Not Worry if You Cannot Find Helpful Strategies on Your Own*

You should not worry if you find it difficult to create your own 'Box Diagram' or if you are unable to find effective strategies on your own. It is very common for those with persisting post-concussion symptoms to need the help of a clinician especially if: it is difficult to stand back from the problems; it is difficult to know where to start because things seem overwhelming; or some of the solutions seem to 'oppose each other'. An example of 'opposing' strategies would be when your diary really helps you with your memory difficulties but robs you of the chance to test out whether your memory is in fact better than you think it is or to challenge negative thoughts about how bad it would be if you do experience memory 'failures'.

Do not hesitate to keep looking for a clinician with experience in mild traumatic brain injury and who can provide the right kind of help for you. Unfortunately, this may involve some persistence as you may not always find the right kind of help the first time around. The right kind of professional can often be a Clinical Neuropsychologist but this will not always be the case.

8. *The Number of Strategies is Limitless so Be Creative!*

Any number of strategies can be used to creatively tackle each of your 'boxes' to make your own 'virtuous cycles' and overcome your PCS to the greatest possible degree. The book only lists the most frequently used ones. Strategies that help any individual are only really limited by their own understanding of what is causing their problems and their imagination to invent ways around them. So be creative!

Final Word!

As I mentioned right at the beginning, I really hope that this book has given you some help, hope and understanding of the highly misunderstood area of MTBI. I would like to wish you all the very best in putting what you have learnt into practice.

Further Reading and Resources

Information on MTBI Designed for Patients and Their Families

R. Morris, *Minor Head Injury* (Nottingham: Headway – the Brain Injury Association, 2009), www.headway.org.uk.

Heart & Mind: Mild Head Injury – A Self-help Guide for Understanding and Managing Post-concussion Symptoms (Salford: Brain and Spinal Injury Centre, n.d.), www.basic charity.org.uk.

Information on MTBI Designed for Clinicians (but with elements helpful to patients)

King, N. S., 'Post–concussion Syndrome: clarity amid the controversy?', *British Journal of Psychiatry*, 183 (2003), 276–8.

Wrightson, P. and D. Gronwall, *Mild Head Injury: A Guide to Management* (Oxford: Oxford University Press, 1999).

Information on Cognitive Behavioural Self-help Strategies for Patients and Families

Robinson publishes the **Overcoming** series of self-help guides to using cognitive behavioural techniques (CBT) with books specifically covering: Anxiety, Stress, Depression, Anger and Irritability, Panic and Agoraphobia, Insomnia and Sleep Problems, Chronic Pain, Worry, Perfectionism, Chronic Fatigue, Health Anxiety and Relationship Problems.

General

Butler, G. and T. Hope, *Manage Your Mind: The Mental Fitness Guide* (Oxford: Oxford University Press, 2007).

www.getselfhelp.co.uk – a free web-based resource with a wide range of CBT self-help material.

Publications by Dr King

Agar, E., P. Kennedy and N. S. King, 'The role of negative cognitive appraisals in PTSD symptoms following spinal cord injuries', *Behavioural & Cognitive Psychotherapy*, 34 (2006), 437–52.

King, N. S., '"Affect without recollection" in post-traumatic stress disorder where head injury causes organic amnesia for the event', *Behavioural & Cognitive Psychotherapy*, 29 (2001), 501–4.

——, 'Emotional, neuropsychological and organic factors: their use in the prediction of post-concussion symptoms after moderate and mild head injuries', *Journal of Neurology, Neurosurgery and Psychiatry*, 61 (1996), 75–81.

——, 'Mild head injury: neuropathology, sequelae, measurement and recovery. A literature review', *British Journal of Clinical Psychology*, 36 (1997), 161–84.

——, 'Perseveration of traumatic memories in PTSD: a cautionary note regarding exposure based psychological treatments for PTSD when head injury and dysexecutive impairment are also present', *Brain Injury*, 16:1 (2002), 65–74.

——, 'The post-concussion syndrome: clarity amid the controversy?', *British Journal of Psychiatry*, 183 (2003), 276–8.

——, 'Post-traumatic stress disorder and head injury as a dual diagnosis: "islands" of memory as a mechanism', *Journal of Neurology, Neurosurgery and Psychiatry*, 62 (1997), 82–4.

——, 'PTSD and head injury: folklore and fact?', *Brain Injury*, 22:1 (2008), 1–5.

——, 'The role of age and gender in permanent post-concussion symptoms after mild head injury: a systematic review of the literature', *Neurorehabilitation*, 34 (2014), 741–8.

——, 'A systematic review of age and gender factors in prolonged post-concussion symptoms after mild head injury', *Brain Injury*, 28:13–14 (2014), 1639–45.

King, N. S., S. Crawford, F. J. Wenden, F. E. Caldwell and D. T. Wade, 'Early prediction of persisting post-concussion symptoms following mild and moderate head injuries', *British Journal of Clinical Psychology*, 38:1 (1999), 15–25.

King, N. S., S. Crawford, F. J. Wenden, N. E. G. Moss and D. T. Wade, 'Interventions and service need following mild and moderate head injury: The Oxford Head Injury Service', *Clinical Rehabilitation*, 11 (1997), 23–7.

——, 'The Rivermead post-concussion symptoms questionnaire – a measure of symptoms commonly experienced after head injury and its reliability', *Journal of Neurology*, 242:9 (1995), 587–92.

King, N. S., S. Crawford, F. J. Wenden, N. E. G. Moss, D. T. Wade and F. E. Caldwell, 'Measurement of post-traumatic amnesia: how reliable is it?', *Journal of Neurology, Neurosurgery and Psychiatry*, 62 (1997), 38–42.

King, N. S. and D. Dean, 'Neuropsychological rehabilitation following acquired brain injury', in H. Beinart, P. Kennedy and S. Llewelyn (eds), *Clinical Psychology in Practice* (Oxford: Blackwell, 2009), 152–63.

King, N. S. and S. Kirwilliam, 'The nature of post-concussion symptoms after mild head injury', *Brain Impairment*, 14:2 (2013), 235–42.

——, 'Permanent post-concussion symptoms following mild head injury', *Brain Injury*, 25:5 (2011), 462–70.

——, 'Factors associated with long-term post-concussion symptoms following mild traumatic brain injury', *Brain Impairment*, 11:2 (2010), 225–6.

King, N. S., J. Pimm and A. Tyerman, 'Enhancing the integration of psychological services for stroke patients through the development of a protocol for Neuropsychology and IAPT Services', *Clinical Psychology Forum*, 255 (2014), 19–25.

King, N. S., 'Providing psychotherapy to people with neuropsychological impairment: complexities and issues raised by the care of "Judith"'. *Pragmatic Case Studies in Psychotherapy*, 11:1 (2015), 21–25.

——, 'Neuropsychological presentation and treatment of traumatic brain injury', in J. Marshall, J. Gurd and U. Kischka (eds), *Handbook of Clinical Neuropsychology* (2nd edition, Oxford: Oxford University Press, 2010).

McGrath, J. and N. S. King, 'Behavioural experiments in acquired brain injury', in J. Bennett-Levy, G. Butler, M. Fennell, A. Hackmann, M. Mueller and D. Westbrook, *The Oxford Guide to Behavioural Experiments in Cognitive Therapy* (Oxford: Oxford University Press, 2004).

Tyerman, A. and N. S. King, 'Interventions for psychological problems after brain injury', in L. M. Goldstein and J. McNeil (eds), *Clinical Neuropsychology: A Practical Guide to Assessment and Management for Clinicians* (2nd edition, Chichester: John Wiley & Sons, 2011).

Tyerman, A. and N. S. King (eds), *Psychological Approaches to Rehabilitation after Traumatic Brain Injury* (Oxford: Blackwell, 2008).

Wade, D. T., S. Crawford, F. J. Wenden, N. S. King and N. E. G. Moss, 'Does routine follow up after head injury help? A randomised controlled trial', *Journal of Neurology, Neurosurgery and Psychiatry*, 62 (1997), 478–84.

Wade, D. T., N. S. King, F. J. Wenden, S. Crawford and F. E. Caldwell, 'Routine follow up after head injury: a second randomised controlled trial', *Journal of Neurology, Neurosurgery and Psychiatry*, 65:2 (1998), 177–83.

Webster, G., A. Daisley and N. S. King, 'Marital and family break up following brain injury: the role of the rehabilitation team', *Brain Injury*, 13:8 (1999), 593–603.

Wenden, F. J., S. Crawford, D. T. Wade, N. S. King and N. E. G. Moss, 'Assault, post-traumatic amnesia and other variables relating to outcome following head injury', *Clinical Rehabilitation*, 12:1 (1998), 53–63.

Index